Evidence Based Medicine in Orthopedic Surgery

Guest Editors

SAFDAR N. KHAN, MD
MARK A. LEE, MD
MUNISH C. GUPTA, MD

ORTHOPEDIC CLINICS
OF NORTH AMERICA

www.orthopedic.theclinics.com

April 2010 • Volume 41 • Number 2

SAUNDERS an imprint of ELSEVIER, Inc.

W.B. SAUNDERS COMPANY
A Division of Elsevier Inc.

1600 John F. Kennedy Blvd. ● Suite 1800 ● Philadelphia, PA 19103-2899.

http://www.orthopedic.theclinics.com

ORTHOPEDIC CLINICS OF NORTH AMERICA Volume 41, Number 2
April 2010 ISSN 0030-5898, ISBN-13: 978-1-4377-1848-5

Editor: Debora Dellapena

Orthopedic Clinics of North America (ISSN 0030-5898) is published quarterly by Elsevier Inc., 360 Park Avenue South, New York, NY 10010-1710. Months of issue are January, April, July, and October. Business and Editorial Offices: 1600 John F. Kennedy Blvd., Suite 1800, Philadelphia, PA 19103-2899. Customer Service Office: 3251 Riverport Lane, Maryland Heights, MO 63043. Periodicals postage paid at New York, NY and additional mailing offices. Subscription prices are $251.00 per year for (US individuals), $458.00 per year for (US institutions), $297.00 per year (Canadian individuals), $549.00 per year (Canadian institutions), $366.00 per year (international individuals), $549.00 per year (international institutions), $126.00 per year (US students), $182.00 per year (Canadian and international students). Foreign air speed delivery is included in all *Clinics* subscription prices. All prices are subject to change without notice. **POSTMASTER:** Send change of address to *Orthopedic Clinics of North America*, **Elsevier Health Sciences Division, Subscription Customer Service, 3251 Riverport Lane, Maryland Heights, MO 63043. Customer Service (orders, claims, online, change of address): Elsevier Health Sciences Division, Subscription Customer Service, 3251 Riverport Lane, Maryland Heights, MO 63043. Tel: 1-800-654-2452 (U.S. and Canada); 314-447-8871 (outside U.S. and Canada). Fax: 314-447-8029. E-mail: journalscustomerservice-usa@elsevier. com (for print support); journalsonlinesupport-usa@elsevier.com (for online support).**

Reprints. For copies of 100 or more, of articles in this publication, please contact the Commercial Reprints Department, Elsevier Inc., 360 Park Avenue South, New York, NY 10010-1710. Tel.: 212-633-3812; Fax: 212-462-1935; E-mail: reprints@elsevier. com.

Orthopedic Clinics of North America is covered in *MEDLINE/PubMed (Index Medicus), Cinahl, Excerpta Medica,* and *Cumulative Index to Nursing and Allied Health Literature.*

Printed and bound by CPI Group (UK) Ltd, Croydon, CR0 4YY

Transferred to Digital Print 2011

Contributors

GUEST EDITORS

SAFDAR N. KHAN, MD
Department of Orthopaedic Surgery, Lawrence
J. Ellison Ambulatory Care Center, University of
California, Davis, Sacramento, California

MARK A. LEE, MD
Department of Orthopaedic Surgery, Lawrence
J. Ellison Ambulatory Care Center, University of
California, Davis, Sacramento, California

MUNISH C. GUPTA, MD
Department of Orthopaedic Surgery, Lawrence
J. Ellison Ambulatory Care Center, University of
California, Davis, Sacramento, California

AUTHORS

DEREK F. AMANATULLAH, MD, PhD
Research Fellow, Department of Orthopaedic
Surgery, University of California Davis Medical
Center, Sacramento, California

ANITA BAGLEY, MPH, PhD
Co-Director, Motion Analysis Laboratory,
Shriners Hospitals for Children, Northern
California; Associate Clinical Professor of
Orthopaedic Surgery, Department of
Orthopaedic Surgery, University
of California, Davis School of Medicine,
Sacramento, California

TIMOTHY C. BEALS, MD
Associate Professor, Department of
Orthopaedics, University of Utah,
Salt Lake City, Utah

SIGURD BERVEN, MD
Associate Professor in Residence,
Department of Orthopaedic Surgery,
University of California, San Francisco,
San Francisco, California

MOHIT BHANDARI, MD, MSc, FRCSC
Canada Research Chair in Musculoskeletal
Trauma; Associate Professor of Orthopaedic
Surgery, Faculty of Health Sciences,
Division of Surgery, Department of Orthopedic
Surgery, McMaster University, Hamilton,
Ontario, Canada

ANGELA J. CAMPBELL, BS
Clinical Research Coordinator,
Department of Orthopaedics, Shriners
Hospitals for Children, Northern California,
Sacramento, California

LEAH Y. CARREON, MD, MSc
Norton Leatherman Spine Center, Louisville,
Kentucky

YEUKKEI CHEUNG, MD
Fellow, Department of Orthopaedic Surgery,
University of California Davis Medical Center,
Sacramento, California

BRETT D. CRIST, MD, FACS
Assistant Professor, Department of
Orthopaedic Surgery, University of Missouri,
Columbia, Missouri

CRAIG J. DELLA VALLE, MD
Attending Orthopaedic Surgeon, Associate
Professor of Orthopaedic Surgery, Rush
University, Chicago, Illinois

PAUL E. DI CESARE, MD
Chair, Department of Orthopaedic Surgery,
University of California Davis Medical Center,
Sacramento, California

JOHN R. DIMAR II, MD
Norton Leatherman Spine Center, Louisville,
Kentucky

ASHISH D. DIWAN, MS, DNB, PhD
Chief, Spine Service, Department
of Orthopedic Surgery, St George
Hospital and Clinical School, University
of New South Wales, Sydney,
Australia

MLADEN DJURASOVIC, MD
Norton Leatherman Spine Center, Louisville,
Kentucky

TANIA A. FERGUSON, MD
Assistant Professor, Department
of Orthopaedic Surgery, Lawrence J.
Ellison Ambulatory Care Center,
University of California, Davis,
Sacramento, California

STEVEN D. GLASSMAN, MD
Norton Leatherman Spine Center, Louisville,
Kentucky

JONATHAN N. GRAUER, MD
Associate Professor, Department of
Orthopaedics and Rehabilitation, Yale
University School of Medicine,
New Haven, Connecticut

BEATE HANSON, MD, PhD
Clinical Assistant Professor and Lecturer
for Cost and Outcome Research,
Department of Health Services, University
of Washington, Seattle, Washington;
AO Foundation, Stettbachstrasse,
Duebendorf, Switzerland

DAVID L. HELFET, MD
Professor of Orthopaedic Surgery,
Weill Cornell Medical College; Director,
Orthopaedic Trauma Service, Hospital
for Special Surgery, New York,
New York

IFTACH HETSRONI, MD
Orthopedic Department, Meir General
Hospital, Sapir Medical Center, Kfar Saba,
Sackler Faculty of Medicine, Tel Aviv
University, Tel Aviv, Israel

THOMAS F. HIGGINS, MD
Associate Professor, Department of
Orthopaedics, University of Utah,
Salt Lake City, Utah

MICHELLE A. JAMES, MD
Chief of Orthopaedic Surgery, Department of
Orthopaedics, Shriners Hospitals for Children,
Northern California; Professor of Clinical
Orthopaedic Surgery, Department of
Orthopaedic Surgery, University of California,
Davis School of Medicine, Sacramento,
California

KOLAWOLE A. JEGEDE, BS
Doris Duke Research Fellow,
Department of Orthopaedics and
Rehabilitation, Yale University School of
Medicine, New Haven, Connecticut

MICHAEL P. KELLY, MD
Resident, Department of Orthopaedic Surgery,
University of California, San Francisco,
San Francisco, California

THOMAS J. KISHEN, MBBS, DNB
Fellow, Spine Service, Department of
Orthopedic Surgery, St George Hospital and
Clinical School, University of New South
Wales, Sydney, Australia

JOSHUA B. KLATT, MD
Assistant Professor, Department of
Orthopaedics, University of Utah, Salt Lake
City, Utah

ERIC KLINEBERG, MD
Assistant Professor; Spine Fellowship
Program Director, Adult and Pediatric
Spinal Surgery, Department of
Orthopaedics, University of California
Davis School of Medicine,
Sacramento, California

JAY R. LIEBERMAN, MD
Attending Orthopaedic Surgeon; Professor
and Chairman, Department of Orthopaedic
Surgery; Director, New England
Musculoskeletal Institute, University of
Connecticut Health Center, Farmington,
Connecticut

JASON A. LOWE, MD
Orthopaedic Trauma Fellow, Department
of Orthopaedic Surgery, Lawrence J. Ellison
Ambulatory Care Center, University of
California, Davis, Sacramento, California

ROBERT G. MARX, MD, FRCSC
Professor, Department of Orthopedic Surgery,
Hospital for Special Surgery, Weill Medical
College of Cornell University, New York,
New York

MICHAEL D. MCKEE, MD, FRCS(C)
Professor, Division of Orthopaedics,
Department of Surgery, St Michael's
Hospital and the University of Toronto,
Toronto, Ontario, Canada

JAMES M. MOK, MD
Fellow, The Spine Institute, Santa Monica,
California

ANTHONY NDU, MD
Department of Orthopaedics and
Rehabilitation, Yale University School of
Medicine, New Haven, Connecticut

SUKHMEET S. PANESAR, BSc (Hons), MBBS
Clinical Advisor to the Medical Director, Patient
Safety Division, National Patient Safety
Agency, London, United Kingdom

MARC J. PHILIPPON, MD
Consultant Surgeon, Steadman Hawkins
Research Foundation, Vail, Colorado

KEITH R. REINHARDT, MD
Resident Physician, Department of
Orthopaedic Surgery, Hospital for
Special Surgery, Weill Medical College
of Cornell University, New York,
New York

NEIL P. SHETH, MD
Adult Reconstructive Fellow, Department
of Orthopaedic Surgery, Rush University,
Midwest Orthopaedics, Chicago,
Illinois

MICHAEL SUK, MD, JD, MPH, FACS
Associate Professor of Orthopaedic
Surgery, University of Florida Health
Science Center; Chief, Division of
Orthopaedic Trauma Surgery, University
of Florida–Shands Jacksonville,
Jacksonville, Florida

ANN VAN HEEST, MD
Professor, Department of Orthopaedic
Surgery, University of Minnesota,
Minneapolis, Minnesota

Contents

Evidence–based medicine integrates clinical expertise, patients' values and preferences, and the best available evidence from the medical literature. Evidence–based orthopedics is a model to assist surgeons to improve the process of asking questions, obtaining relevant information efficiently, and making informed decisions with patients. With an increasing appreciation for higher levels of evidence, orthopedic surgeons should move away from lower forms of evidence. The adoption of randomized trials and high-quality prospective studies to guide patient care requires 2 prerequisites: (1) greater appreciation for the conduct of randomized trials in orthopedics and (2) improved education and training in evidence-based methodologies in surgery.

The promise of evidence-based medicine is to integrate the highest levels of clinical data with patient outcomes. After framing the question and identifying appropriate studies, evaluating their relevance to clinical practice is highly dependent on the instruments and measures selected to demonstrate outcomes. Currently, there are hundreds of outcomes measures available in the orthopedic literature evaluating these treatments, and it is not uncommon for different measures to produce conflicting results. Consequently, the ability to evaluate an outcomes measure is critical in determining the value of a specific treatment intervention. Similarly, selecting the appropriate outcomes measure for research or clinical purposes is an important decision that may have far reaching implications on reimbursement, surgeon reputation, and patient treatment success. Evidence-based orthopedic surgery is indeed possible, but demands a detailed understanding of why appropriate outcomes selection is important, the difference between clinician-based and patient-reported outcomes (PROs), and potential future directions in orthopedics outcomes research.

The concept of evidence-based medicine has gained broad support in the medical community, because clinical decisions based on information from rigorous scientific study are most likely to provide optimal care. Researchers attempt to answer clinical questions using either observational studies or randomized controlled trials (RCTs). Observational studies currently dominate the surgical literature but provide a level of evidence inferior to RCTs. RCTs are ethically grounded in clinical equipoise and may further reduce the potential for bias or other confounding factors by blinding. This article discusses the barriers to implementation of surgical RCTs.

Dynamic stabilization of the spine has applications in cervical and lumbar degenerative disease and in thoracolumbar trauma. There is little evidence to support the use of dynamic cervical plates rather than rigid anterior cervical fixation. Evidence to support the use of dynamic constructs for fusion in the lumbar spine is also limited. Fusion rates, implant loosening, and failure are significant concerns that limit the adoption of current devices. This article provides a synopsis of the literature on human subjects. There is a need for high-quality evidence for interventions for spinal pathology. An evidence-based approach to the management of spinal disorders will require ongoing assessment of clinical outcomes and comparison of effectiveness between alternatives.

Lumbar disc herniations are common clinical entities that may cause lumbar-related symptoms. The spectrum of treatment options is geared toward a patient's clinical presentation and ranges from nothing to surgical intervention. Many lumbar disc herniations cause no significant symptoms. In studies of asymptomatic individuals who have never experienced lumbar-related symptoms, 30% have been reported to have major abnormality on magnetic resonance imaging. The mainstay of treatment of patients with symptomatic disc herniations is accepted to be nonoperative (as long as there are no acute or progressive neurologic deficits); this includes medications, physical therapy, and potentially lumbar injection. For patients with symptomatic disc herniations who fail to respond appropriately to conservative measures, surgical intervention may be considered. For this population, lumbar discectomy is considered to be a good option.

Clavicle fractures are common, and they comprise close to 3% of all fractures seen in fracture clinics. Midshaft fractures account for approximately 80% of all clavicle fractures and are the focus of this article. In carefully selected cases primary plate fixation of displaced midshaft clavicle fractures improves outcome, results in earlier return to function, and reduces the nonunion and symptomatic malunion rate significantly compared with nonoperative treatment.

Lower Extremity Assessment Project (LEAP) study set out to answer many of the questions surrounding the decision of whether to amputate or salvage limbs in the setting of severe lower extremity trauma. A National Institutes of Health–funded, multicenter, prospective observational study, the LEAP study represented a milestone in orthopedic trauma research, and perhaps in orthopedics. The LEAP study attempted to define the characteristics of the individuals who sustained these injuries, the characteristics of their environment, the variables of the physical aspects of their injury, the secondary medical and mental conditions that arose from their injury and treatment, their ultimate functional status, and their general health. In the realm of evidence-based medicine, the LEAP studies provided a wealth of data, but still failed to completely determine treatment at the onset of severe lower extremity trauma.

David L. Helfet, Michael Suk, and Beate Hanson

The Study to Prospectively evaluate Reamed Intramedullary Nails in Tibial fractures (SPRINT) was a randomized controlled trial to evaluate rates of reoperation and complications resulting from reamed versus unreamed intramedullary nailing for the treatment of tibial shaft fractures. The trial found a possible benefit for reamed intramedullary nailing in patients with closed tibial fractures, but no difference was found between the 2 approaches in patients with open fractures. This article is a review and critique of the methodology used in the SPRINT trial. Numerous aspects of the trial's design served to greatly reduce the potential bias, producing sound and reliable results. Overall, the SPRINT trial should provide recommendations for change in clinical practice and also set a benchmark for the conduct of randomized controlled trials in orthopedic surgery.

Keith R. Reinhardt, Iftach Hetsroni, and Robert G. Marx

Tear of the anterior cruciate ligament (ACL) is the most common ligamentous injury of the knee. Reconstructing this ligament is often required to restore functional stability of the knee. Many graft options are available for ACL reconstruction, including different autograft and allograft tissues. Autografts include bone-patellar tendon-bone composites (PT), combined semitendinosus and gracilis hamstring tendons (HT), and quadriceps tendon. Allograft options include the same types of tendons harvested from donors, in addition to Achilles and tibialis tendons. Tissue-engineered anterior cruciate grafts are not yet available for clinical use, but may become a feasible alternative in the future. The purpose of this systematic review is to assess whether one of the popular grafts (PT and HT) is preferable for reconstructing the ACL. For this objective, the authors selected only true level I studies that compared these graft choices in functional clinical outcomes, failure rates, and other objective parameters following reconstruction of the ACL. In addition, this review discusses mechanical considerations related to different allograft tissues.

Derek F. Amanatullah, Yeukkei Cheung, and Paul E. Di Cesare

Hip resurfacing arthroplasty has reemerged as a valid reconstruction option for the osteoarthritic hip. Patient selection is critical for excellent surgical outcomes, especially when compared with total hip arthroplasty. However, concerns regarding surgical technique and postsurgical complications persist. The authors review the evidence for surgical technique, outcomes, and complications related to modern metal-on-metal hip resurfacing arthroplasty.

Neil P. Sheth, Jay R. Lieberman, and Craig J. Della Valle

Deep venous thrombosis (DVT) is the end result of a complex interaction of events including the activation of the clotting cascade in conjunction with platelet aggregation. Patients undergoing major lower extremity orthopedic surgery, especially total joint arthroplasty (TJA), are at high risk for developing a postoperative DVT or a subsequent pulmonary embolus. Venous thromboembolic (VTE) prophylaxis, most commonly pharmacologic prophylaxis, has become the standard of care for patients undergoing elective TJA. However, the controversy between the efficacy of VTE prophylaxis and the increased risk for bleeding in the postoperative period continues to exist. This review addresses the controversy underlying VTE prophylaxis by outlining 2 guidelines and demonstrating the pros and cons of different DVT prophylaxis regimens based on the available evidence-based literature.

Orthopedic Clinics of North America

THE CLINICS ARE NOW AVAILABLE ONLINE!

Access your subscription at:
www.theclinics.com

Preface

Evidence–Based Medicine in Orthopedic Surgery

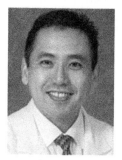 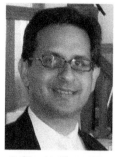 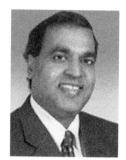

Mark A. Lee, MD   Safdar N. Khan, MD   Munish C. Gupta, MD

Guest Editors

The principles of evidence-based medicine have been available to us since "The Canon of Medicine" was completed in 1025 by Avicenna. The application of best available evidence to contemporary clinical decision making is not a new one—however, our appreciation of the impact these concepts have on patient care have recently become a subject of great interest.

The current issue of the *Orthopedic Clinics of North America* is dedicated to understanding the application of evidence-based medicine as it relates to the art and science of orthopedic surgery. Contemporary readers have unparalleled access to many publications explaining the core principles of evidence-based research in orthopedic surgery; however, we (and an exceptional cadre of contributing authors) have focused specifically on an evaluation of the quality of evidence in several controversial areas in orthopedic surgery. This list is far from conclusive; however, our hope is that readers will use these articles and their methodology as a template for evidence-based treatment recommendations.

We would like to congratulate and thank all of our authors for their generous efforts and thoughtful contributions to this compilation. Finally, we would like to acknowledge the vision, dedication, and perseverance of Deb Dellapena at Elsevier, who has made developing this volume an immense pleasure.

Safdar N. Khan, MD
Department of Orthopaedic Surgery
Lawrence J. Ellison Ambulatory Care Center
University of California, Davis
4860 Y Street, Suite 1700
Sacramento, CA 95817, USA

Mark A. Lee, MD
Department of Orthopaedic Surgery
Lawrence J. Ellison Ambulatory Care Center
University of California, Davis
4860 Y Street, Suite 1700
Sacramento, CA 95817, USA

Munish C. Gupta, MD
Department of Orthopaedic Surgery
Lawrence J. Ellison Ambulatory Care Center
University of California, Davis
4860 Y Street, Suite 1700
Sacramento, CA 95817, USA

E-mail addresses:
safdar.khan@ucdmc.ucdavis.edu (S.N. Khan)
mark.lee@ucdmc.ucdavis.edu (M.A. Lee)
munish.gupta@ucdmc.ucdavis.edu (M.C. Gupta)

doi:10.1016/j.ocl.2010.03.003
0030-5898/10/$ – see front matter

orthopedic.theclinics.com

Principles of Evidence-Based Medicine

Sukhmeet S. Panesar, BSc (Hons), MBBS[a],
Marc J. Philippon, MD[b], Mohit Bhandari, MD, MSc, FRCSC[c],*

KEYWORDS

- Evidence-based medicine • Orthopedics
- Statistics • Evidence synthesis

The origins of what is currently known as evidence-based medicine (EBM) go as far back as the seventeenth century, when it was observed that patients who received bleeding as part of their treatment of cholera had a much higher mortality rate than those who were not treated in the same manner.[1] It has only been recently that EBM has seen an exponential increase in its adoption, and indeed the development of EBM has been heralded as one of the top medical milestones over the last 160 years.[2] Although definitions vary, EBM integrates clinical expertise, patients' values and preferences, and the best available evidence from the medical literature.[3] In other words, as suggested by Sackett and colleagues,[4] "Evidence based medicine is the conscientious, explicit, and judicious use of current best evidence in making decisions about the care of individual patients."

Historically, surgical decisions have largely been based on personal experience and recommendations from surgical authorities. In contrast to internal medicine, trials of surgical techniques and technologies have unique challenges and have, therefore, been slow to permeate the surgical literature. In addition, regulatory bodies have imposed less stringent controls on the validation of these technologies. As such, most surgical practice is based on lower levels of evidence.[5] The proportion of systematic reviews and randomized controlled trials (RCTs) in leading surgical journals stands at 5%.[6]

Regardless of the overall number of trials in surgery, it is extremely difficult for practicing surgeons to keep abreast of critical evidence, given the large number of surgical articles published monthly. Haynes stipulates that doctors need to read approximately 20 articles a day to keep up to date in their field.[7]

Surgery is an exponentially growing specialty with 234 million operations performed globally in a year.[8] Of these, 64 million are performed in the United States, and health care accounts for one-sixth of the economy.[9] Furthermore, Internet-savvy patients who want the best in diagnostics and therapies demand evidence-based practice. The onus is on surgeons to provide high-quality evidence and institute best practices.

EVIDENCE-BASED ORTHOPEDICS

Current estimates suggest that less than 5% of the orthopedic literature represents randomized trials, although this has been steadily increasing.[10] However, even the quality of reporting in RCTs is highly variable. Complete reporting of allocation concealment, details of blinding in follow-up, and surgical expertise in trial reports have been uncommon.[11]

Although many orthopedic journals (eg, *Journal of Bone and Joint Surgery*, *Clinical Orthopaedics and Related Research*, *Acta Orthopaedica*, *Journal of Orthopaedic Trauma*, and *Orthopedic Clinics of North America*) have adopted evidence-based approaches to reporting clinical research, there remain considerable opportunities to improve

[a] Patient Safety Division, National Patient Safety Agency, 4-8 Maple Street, W1T 5HD, London, UK
[b] Steadman Hawkins Research Foundation, 181 West Meadow Drive, Suite 1000, Vail, CO 81657, USA
[c] Faculty of Health Sciences, Division of Surgery, Department of Orthopedic Surgery, McMaster University, 293 Wellington Street North, Suite 110, Hamilton, Ontario L8S 4L8, Canada
* Corresponding author.
E-mail address: bhandam@mcmaster.ca

Orthop Clin N Am 41 (2010) 131–138
doi:10.1016/j.ocl.2009.12.001

processes. Providing additional evidence-based resources and education for readers is a key first step.

GRADING OF EVIDENCE

The Oxford Center for Evidence Based Medicine has come up with a detailed hierarchy of evidence, as illustrated in **Fig. 1**.[12] The highest form of evidence remains a systematic review of homogeneous RCTs. A further step in grading of evidence is GRADE (Grades of Recommendation, Assessment, Development, and Evaluation). GRADE allows for a comprehensive, explicit, and transparent methodology for grading the quality of evidence and strength of recommendations about the management of patients.[13]

Surgeons may believe that they are at risk of losing their autonomy with the proliferation of evidence-based guidelines. In today's approach to using information, surgeons have to consider a change from a traditional paradigm of "this is how we have always done it" toward the application of current best evidence practices based on reliable and valid information sources. At the heart of EBM lies the amalgamation of individual clinical expertise, patient preferences, and best available evidence.[14]

CHALLENGES OF CONDUCTING RCTS IN SURGERY

Proponents of EBM have always been cautious about the generalizability of results to a specific population or setting. Several problems in conducting RCTs in surgery have been reported. These problems include a general lack of knowledge, tendency to rigorously defend historically performed techniques, learning curve issues (seniority usually results in better outcomes), difficulty in blinding, and ethical considerations.[15] One solution to overcome known biases in surgical trials is the expertise-based RCT. In this type of trial, a surgeon with expertise in one of the procedures being evaluated is paired with a surgeon with expertise in the other procedure who should ideally be from the same institution. Subjects are randomized to treatments and treated by a surgeon who is an "expert" in the procedure. This study overcomes some of the challenges associated with traditional orthopedic RCTs, including the caveat that surgeons who wish to participate in traditional RCTs must be willing to perform both techniques, and that a lack of expertise or belief in one of the interventions under evaluation may undermine the validity and applicability of the results.[16] A recent survey of orthopedic surgeons found that most would consider this type of study design as it may decrease the likelihood of procedural crossovers and enhance validity because, unlike the conventional RCT, there is a low likelihood of differential expertise bias.[17] Furthermore, positive steps are being made with the advent of larger multicenter trials in orthopedic surgery.[18]

THE VALUE OF OBSERVATIONAL STUDIES WHEN NO RCTS EXIST

A significant proportion of the surgical literature finds its form as observational studies. It must be remembered that much of the research into the cause of diseases relies on cohort, case-control, or cross-sectional studies. Observational studies can generate significant hypotheses and have a role in delineating the harms and benefits of interventions. To ensure the robustness of reporting observational studies, the STROBE statement was created. The STROBE guidelines aim to assist investigators when writing up analytical observational studies, to support editors and reviewers when considering such articles for publication, and to help readers when critically appraising published articles.[19]

LEARNING THE "NEW" LANGUAGE OF EBM

EBM practitioners do not have to become statisticians; however, they do need to understand key concepts and terminology to optimize their experiences.

Relative Risk, Odds Ratios, and Number Needed to Treat

If the end point of a study is binary or dichotomous, such as mortality or no mortality, then the odds ratio (OR) or relative risk or risk ratio (RR) can be calculated. The OR is the probability that a particular event will occur to the probability that it will not occur, and can be any number between zero and infinity. Risk describes the probability with which a health outcome (usually an adverse event) will occur. Measures of relative effect express the outcome in one group relative to that in the other. For treatments that increase the chances of events, the OR will be larger than the RR, so the tendency will be to misinterpret the findings in the form of an overestimation of treatment effect. OR is for case-controlled studies and RR is for cohort studies. Absolute measures, such as the absolute risk reduction or the number of patients needed to be treated (NNT) to prevent one event, are more helpful when applying results in clinical practice. The NNT can be calculated as 1/risk difference (RD).[20]

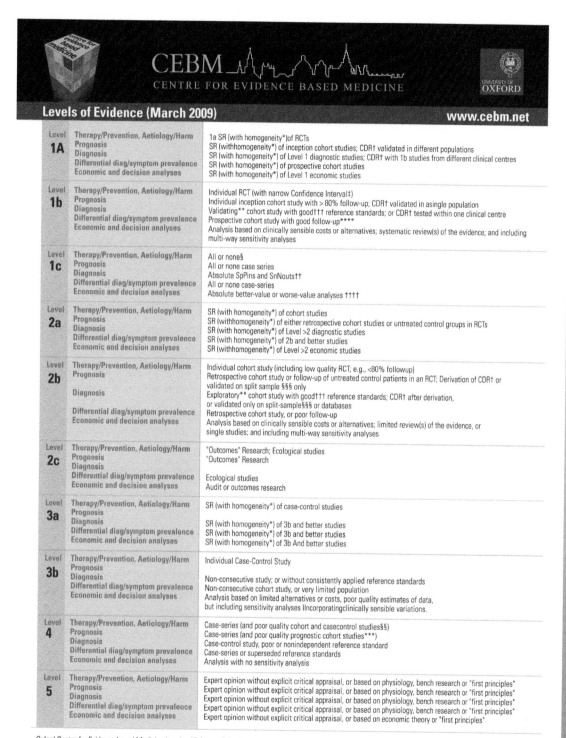

Fig. 1. Levels of evidence. (*From* Oxford Centre for Evidence-Based Medicine. Available at: http://www.cebm.net/index.aspx?o=1025. Accessed August 5, 2009; with permission.)

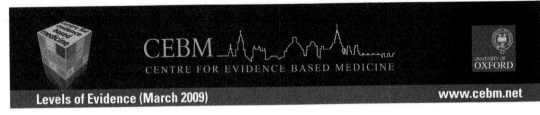

Levels of Evidence (March 2009)

www.cebm.net

NOTES

Users can add a minus-sign "-" to denote the level of that fails to provide a conclusive answer because:

EITHER   a single result with a wide Confidence Interval

OR   a Systematic Review with troublesome heterogeneity.

Such evidence is inconclusive, and therefore can only generate Grade D recommendations.

*	By homogeneity we mean a systematic review that is free of worrisome variations (heterogeneity) in the directions and degrees of results between individual studies. Not all systematic reviews with statistically significant heterogeneity need be worrisome, and not all worrisome heterogeneity need be statistically significant. As noted above, studies displaying worrisome heterogeneity should be tagged with a "-" at the end of their designated level.
†	Clinical Decision Rule. (These are algorithms or scoring systems that lead to a prognostic estimation or a diagnostic category.)
‡	See note above for advice on how to understand, rate and use trials or other studies with wide confidence intervals.
§	Met when all patients died before the Rx became available, but some now survive on it; or when some patients died before the Rx became available, but none now die on it.
§§	By poor quality cohort study we mean one that failed to clearly define comparison groups and/or failed to measure exposures and outcomes in the same (preferably blinded), objective way in both exposed and nonexposed individuals and/or failed to identify or appropriately control known confounders and/or failed to carry out a sufficiently long and complete follow-up of patients. By poor quality case-control study we mean one that failed to clearly define comparison groups and/or failed to measure exposures and outcomes in the same (preferably blinded), objective way in both cases and controls and/or failed to identify or appropriately control known confounders.
§§§	Split-sample validation is achieved by collecting all the information in a single tranche, then artificially dividing this into "derivation" and "validation" samples.
††	An "Absolute SpPin" is a diagnostic finding whose Specificity is so high that a Positive result rules-in the diagnosis. An "Absolute SnNout" is a diagnostic finding whose Sensitivity is so high that a Negative result rules out the diagnosis.
‡‡	Good, better, bad and worse refer to the comparisons between treatments in terms of their clinical risks and benefits.
†††	Good reference standards are independent of the test, and applied blindly or objectively to applied to all patients. Poor reference standards are haphazardly applied, but still independent of the test. Use of a non-independent reference standard (where the 'test' is included in the 'reference', or where the 'testing' affects the 'reference') implies a level 4 study.
††††	Better-value treatments are clearly as good but cheaper, or better at the same or reduced cost. Worse-value treatments are as good and more expensive, or worse and the equally or more expensive.
**	Validating studies test the quality of a specific diagnostic test, based on prior evidence. An exploratory study collects information and trawls the data (e.g. using a regression analysis) to find which factors are 'significant'.
***	By poor quality prognostic cohort study we mean one in which sampling was biased in favour of patients who already had the target outcome, or the measurement of outcomes was accomplished in <80% of study patients, or outcomes were determined in an unblinded, non-objective way, or there was no correction for confounding factors.
****	Good follow-up in a differential diagnosis study is >80%, with adequate time for alternative diagnoses to emerge (for example 1-6 months acute, 1 - 5 years chronic)

Grades of Recommendation

A	consistent level 1 studies
B	consistent level 2 or 3 studies or extrapolations from level 1 studies
C	level 4 studies or extrapolations from level 2 or 3 studies
D	level 5 evidence or troublingly inconsistent or inconclusive studies of any level

"Extrapolations" are where data is used in a situation that has potentially clinically important differences than the original study situation.

Oxford Centre for Evidence-based Medicine Levels of Evidence (March 2009)
(for definitions of terms used see glossary at http://www.cebm.net/?o=1116)

Produced by Bob Phillips, Chris Ball, Dave Sackett, Doug Badenoch, Sharon Straus, Brian Haynes, Martin Dawes since November 1998. Updated by Jeremy Howick March 2009.

Fig. 1. (*continued*)

Let us take the example shown in **Table 1**, which is a hypothetical dataset from a cohort of patients who had cement inserted after hemiarthroplasty and who were compared with a matched sample of patients who did not have any cement inserted during hemiarthroplasty.

The absolute risk reduction (ARR), which is the difference in risk between the control group and the intervention group, is calculated as $ARR = [(c/(c + d) - a/(a + b))] \times 100\% = [(12/(12 + 60)) - (3/(3 + 50))] \times 100\% = 11\%$

The relative risk (RR) is the ratio of risk in the intervention (Y) to the risk in the control group (X) and as such $RR = Y/X = (a/(a + b))/(c/(c + d)) = (3/(3 + 50))/12/(12 + 60) = 0.35$

The relative risk reduction (RRR) is the percentage reduction in risk in the intervention compared with the control group, so $RRR = 1 - RR = (1 - X/Y) \times 100\% = 65\%$

$NNT - 1/ARR = 1/14.1\% = 9$.

Bias

All research studies are prone to a degree of bias. Bias is the inclusion of a nonrandom systematic error in the design of a study. Several forms of bias exist, including patient selection (selection and membership bias), study performance (performance and information bias), patient follow-up (nonresponder and transfer bias), and outcome determination (detection, recall, acceptability, and interviewer bias). Frequent biases in the orthopedic literature include selection bias, when dissimilar groups are compared; nonresponder bias, when the follow-up rate is low; and interviewer bias, when the investigator determines the outcome.[21] Another key form of bias is publication bias, which refers to the greater likelihood of studies with positive results being published.[22] The exclusion of studies for being small in size, publishing negative results or otherwise can bias the results. Even though a recent study found no evidence of publication bias in the orthopedics literature, it is important that orthopedic surgeons know about the findings of studies with a negative or neutral result.[23]

P Values and Confidence Intervals

A P value is the probability that results as extreme as or more so than those observed would occur if the null hypothesis was true and the experiments were repeated over and over. Confidence intervals are a range of 2 values within which it is probable that the true value lies for the entire population of patients from which the study patients were selected.[24] It has already been shown that P values, when significant, unduly influence the perceptions of orthopedic surgeons regarding the importance of study results.[25] It is worth noting that a strict cut-off point such as $P<.05$ is arbitrary, and as such, there is a tendency to make better use of confidence intervals. P values give no information about the strength of the association, and the P value may be statistically significant without the results being clinically important. Conversely, 95% confidence intervals reveal the magnitude of differences and the precision of measurement.[21]

PRACTICING EBM

Surgeons lacking proficiency in EBM may be misled by the orthopedic literature. The onus is on the orthopedic surgeon to develop a robust method to appraise the evidence. There are 5 main steps involved in the practice of EBM. This approach was suggested by the Sicily statement and have a robust evidence base surrounding their use[26]:

Asking a Focused Question

Asking a focused question helps to translate uncertainty into an answerable question. To achieve its goal the question must include the following components:

1. The patient or the problem being addressed (eg, "in patients with femoral neck fractures...")
2. The intervention or exposure being considered (eg, "....would perform arthroplasty...")

Table 1
Hypothetical data on mortality after cemented versus uncemented hemiarthroplasty

	Mortality After Hemiarthroplasty	
	+	−
Bone cement inserted (Y)	3 (a)	50 (b)
No cement inserted (X)	12 (c)	60 (d)

3. The comparison intervention or exposure (eg, ".....be more efficacious than internal fixation...")
4. The clinical outcomes of interest (eg, "...and lead to lower mortality, faster mobilization, and decreased rates of revision...").

These components can be remembered by the PICO (patient, population, problem, intervention, comparison, and outcome) mnemonic as shown in **Fig. 2**.[24]

Finding the Evidence

Finding the evidence involves systematically retrieving the best evidence available. There are several sources of information other than textbooks which are still frequently used by orthopedic surgeons, and the information is often out of date by the time a textbook has gone to press.[14] Medical databases can be a useful source of information. Studies are usually indexed into searchable fields (such as author, title, source, or subject). One popular database is Medline/PubMed. PubMed is part of the US National Library of Medicine (NLM) that includes over 19 million citations from MEDLINE and other life science journals for biomedical articles dating back to 1948. MEDLINE is the largest component of PubMed. Approximately 5200 journals published in the United States and more than 80 other countries have been selected and are currently indexed for MEDLINE. A distinctive feature of MEDLINE is that the records are indexed with NLM's controlled vocabulary, the Medical Subject Headings.[27]

In addition to being able to navigate popular databases such as Medline or Embase, orthopedic surgeons should familiarize themselves with other sources of information such as Cumulative Index to Nursing and Allied Health Literature (CINAHL), Educational Resources Information Center (ERIC), PsycInfo, Public Affairs Information Service (PAIS) International, Bandolier, BestBETS, and the Cochrane collaboration, to name but a few.

Critical Appraisal

Critical appraisal is a crucial step that involves testing the evidence for validity, clinical relevance, and applicability of a study. Most surgical evidence does not come in the form of meta-analyses or indeed RCTs. When faced with the latest paper comparing an implant X versus implant Y or conservative management, the reader must consider a few questions. Both observational studies and RCTs have a set of questions, which help in the critical appraisal of the article, and which must resonate in the mind of the orthopedic surgeon. These questions are shown in **Table 2**.[28,29]

Making a Decision

Once all the information has been obtained and appraised, high-quality data should be applied to the clinical situation weighing the benefits and limitations of applying the therapy.

Evaluating Performance

Once a change has been made to clinical practice, it must be audited and assessed to ascertain the true merits and demerits of the change. This process allows for a continuous cycle of self-improvement. Clinical audit has been defined as "A quality improvement process that seeks to improve patient care and outcomes through systematic review of care against explicit criteria and the implementation of change. Aspects of the structure, processes, and outcomes of care are selected and systematically evaluated against explicit criteria. Where indicated, changes are implemented at an individual, team, or service level and further monitoring is used to confirm improvement in health care delivery."[30]

PICO clinical patient-oriented questions	
P Patient Population Problem	Describe your patient group.
I Intervention	Which main intervention, prognostic factor, or exposure is being considered?
C Comparison	What is the main alternative treatment to compare to I (intervention)?
O Outcome	What result can be expected from the intervention?
	What outcome is relevant to you and your patient?
	What type of question are you asking?
	What would be the best study design/methodology?

Fig. 2. The "PICO" questionnaire. (From Poolman RW, Kerkhoffs GM, Struijs PA, et al. Don't be misled by the orthopedic literature: tips for critical appraisal. Acta Orthop 2007;78(2):163; with permission.)

Table 2
A practical approach to critically appraising a study

Type of Study	Steps	Specific Details
Observational	Primary survey	• Did the study have a representative sample of patients? • Was a homogeneous set of patients selected? Were any subgroups selected?
	Secondary survey	• Was there adequate follow-up of the patients? • Did the authors use objective and unbiased outcome criteria?
	Results	• Was adequate statistical methodology used to achieve robust outcomes? • What is the precision of the estimates of likelihood?
	My practice	• Are the results applicable to my practice? • Are the likely treatment benefits worth the potential harm and costs?
RCTs	Validity	• Were the patients similar in the different treatment arms of the study? • Was randomization adequate, and were patients analyzed in the groups to which they were randomized? • How blinded were the studies in terms of both design and analysis? • Were patients adequately followed up?
	Results	• How large was the treatment effect? • How precise was the estimate of the treatment effect?
	My practice	• Are the results applicable to my practice? • Are the likely treatment benefits worth the potential harm and costs?

Adapted from Bhandari M, Guyatt GH, Swiontkowski MF. User's guide to the orthopaedic literature: how to use an article about a surgical therapy. J Bone Joint Surg Am 2001;83-A(6):917; with permission.

WHY BOTHER WITH EBM?

Evidence-based orthopedics is a model to assist surgeons to improve the process of asking questions, obtaining relevant information efficiently, and making informed decisions with patients. With an increasing appreciation for higher levels of evidence, orthopedic surgeons should move away from lower forms of evidence. The adoption of randomized trials and high-quality prospective studies to guide patient care requires 2 prerequisites: (1) greater appreciation for the conduct of randomized trials in orthopedics and (2) improved education and training in evidence-based methodologies in surgery.

REFERENCES

1. Strauss SE, McAlister FA. Evidence-based medicine: past, present, and future. Ann R Coll Physicians Surg Can 1999;32:260–4.
2. Bhandari M. Evidence-based medicine: why bother? Arthroscopy 2009;25(3):296–7.
3. Guyatt GH, Sackett DL, Sinclair JC, et al. Users' guides to the medical literature. IX. A method for grading health care recommendations. Evidence-Based Medicine Working Group. JAMA 1995; 274(22):1800–4.
4. Sackett DL, Rosenberg WM, Gray JA, et al. Evidence based medicine: what it is and what it isn't. BMJ 1996; 312(7023):71–2.
5. Jones RS, Richards K. Office of Evidence-Based Surgery charts course for improved system of care. Bull Am Coll Surg 2003;88(4):11–21.
6. Panesar SS, Thakrar R, Athanasiou T, et al. Comparison of reports of randomized controlled trials and systematic reviews in surgical journals: literature review. J R Soc Med 2006;99(9):470–2.
7. Haynes RB. Where's the meat in clinical journals? ACP J Club 1993;119:A23–4.
8. Weiser TG, Regenbogen SE, Thompson K, et al. An estimation of the global volume of surgery: a modelling strategy based on available data. Lancet 2008; 372(9633):139–44.
9. Gawande A. Getting there from here: how should Obama reform health care? New Yorker 2009;1: 26–33.
10. Sung J, Siegel J, Tornetta P, et al. The orthopaedic trauma literature: an evaluation of statistically significant findings in orthopaedic trauma randomized trials. BMC Musculoskelet Disord 2008;9:14.

11. Chan S, Bhandari M. The quality of reporting of orthopaedic randomized trials with use of a checklist for nonpharmacological therapies. J Bone Joint Surg Am 2007;89(9):1970–8.

12. Oxford Centre for Evidence Based Medicine. Available at: http://www.cebm.net/index.aspx?o=1025. Accessed August 5, 2009.

13. Brozek JL, Akl EA, Alonso-Coello P, et al. Grading quality of evidence and strength of recommendations in clinical practice guidelines. Part 1 of 3. An overview of the GRADE approach and grading quality of evidence about interventions. Allergy 2009;64(5):669–77.

14. Poolman RW, Petrisor BA, Marti RK, et al. Misconceptions about practicing evidence-based orthopedic surgery. Acta Orthop 2007;78(1):2–11.

15. McCulloch P, Taylor I, Sasako M, et al. Randomised trials in surgery: problems and possible solutions. BMJ 2002;324(7351):1448–51.

16. Devereaux PJ, Bhandari M, Clarke M, et al. Need for expertise based randomised controlled trials. BMJ 2005;330:88.

17. Bednarska E, Bryant D, Devereaux PJ, et al. Orthopaedic surgeons prefer to participate in expertise-based randomized trials. Clin Orthop Relat Res 2008;466(7):1734–44.

18. Sprague S, Matta JM, Bhandari M. Multicenter collaboration in observational research: improving generalizability and efficiency. J Bone Joint Surg Am 2009;91(Suppl 3):80–6.

19. von Elm E, Altman DG, Egger M, et al. The Strengthening the Reporting of Observational Studies in Epidemiology (STROBE) statement: guidelines for reporting observational studies. Lancet 2007; 370(9596):1453–7.

20. Measures of relative effect: the risk ratio and odds ratio. In: Higgins JPT, Green S, editors. Cochrane Handbook for Systematic Reviews of Interventions, version 5.0.2 [updated September 2009]. The Cochrane Collaboration, 2009. Available at: www.cochrane-handbook.org. Accessed January 22, 2010.

21. Kocher MS, Zurakowski D. Clinical epidemiology and biostatistics: a primer for orthopaedic surgeons. J Bone Joint Surg Am 2004;86(3):607–20.

22. Easterbrook PJ, Berlin JA, Gopalan R, et al. Publication bias in clinical research. Lancet 1991; 337(8746):867–72.

23. Okike K, Kocher MS, Mehlman CT, et al. Publication bias in orthopaedic research: an analysis of scientific factors associated with publication in the Journal of Bone and Joint Surgery (American Volume). J Bone Joint Surg Am 2008;90(3):595–601.

24. Poolman RW, Kerkhoffs GM, Struijs PA, et al. Don't be misled by the orthopedic literature: tips for critical appraisal. Acta Orthop 2007;78(2):162–71.

25. Bhandari M, Tornetta P 3rd, Ellis T, et al. Hierarchy of evidence: differences in results between non-randomized studies and randomized trials in patients with femoral neck fractures. Arch Orthop Trauma Surg 2004;124(1):10–6.

26. Dawes M, Summerskill W, Glasziou P, et al. Sicily statement on evidence based practice. BMC Med Educ 2005;5(1):1.

27. United Stated National Library of Medicine, National Institutes of Health. What is the difference between PubMed and MEDLINE? Available at: http://www.nlm.nih.gov/pubs/factsheets/dif_med_pub.html. Accessed January 22, 2010.

28. Bhandari M, Guyatt GH, Swiontkowski MF. User's guide to the orthopaedic literature: how to use an article about a surgical therapy. J Bone Joint Surg Am 2001;83(6):916–26.

29. Jones A, Dollery W. Admission not needs for uncomplicated sternal fractures. BESTBets. Available at: http://www.bestbets.org/bets/bet.php?id=5. Accessed January 22, 2010.

30. National Institute of Health and Clinical Excellence (NICE). Principles for best practice in clinical audit. Available at: http://www.nice.org.uk/media/796/23/BestPracticeClinicalAudit.pdf. Accessed January 22, 2010.

Evidence-Based Orthopedic Surgery: Is It Possible?

Michael Suk, MD, JD, MPH[a,b,]*, Beate Hanson, MD, PhD[c,d], David L. Helfet, MD[e,f]

KEYWORDS

- Evidence-based medicine • Evidence-based orthopedics
- Outcomes research

In recent years, evidence-based medicine has evolved from an outpost of clinical research to the mainstream of clinical practice. Broadly defined as "the integration of clinical expertise with the best available clinical evidence and patients' values,"[1] its scope demands an understanding of the hierarchy of evidence with a deliberate focus on a patient's subjective commentary. Conceptually, the principles of evidence-based medicine are well accepted and they provide the means to critically evaluate clinical research.[2]

When applied to the treatment of musculoskeletal conditions, evidence-based medicine is often referred to as evidence-based orthopedics.[3] Similar to evidence-based medicine, evidence-based orthopedics involves 4 primary steps: (1) formulating a clear question based on the patient's problem, (2) identifying relevant studies from the literature, (3) critically appraising the validity and usefulness of the identified studies, and (4) applying the findings in clinical practice.[4]

Evaluation of the usefulness of evidence-based orthopedics has traditionally been focused on question development, defining levels of evidence for the purpose of education, and structuring a common language between readers. The PICO format (Patients, Interventions, Comparisons, and Outcomes of interest) is commonly used to formulate focused questions to be answered, followed by a review of all pertinent studies and evaluations relevant to their position in the hierarchy of evidence.[5]

Since January 2003, all clinical scientific articles published in the *Journal of Bone and Joint Surgery* (American Volume) have included a level-of-evidence rating.[6] As a result of this rating, most orthopedic surgeons today are familiar with the concepts embodied by evidence-based medicine, yet remain skeptical about its relevance in their own clinical practice. In 2007, attendees at the Annual Meeting of the American Orthopaedic Association (AOA) were asked, "Why is evidence-based medicine not universally embraced by the practicing orthopedic surgeon in clinical decision making?" Although roughly 10% indicated a lack of understanding of evidence-based medicine, 66% cited a lack of appropriate clinical evidence relevant to one's practice.[7] Overcoming this barrier may be evidence-based medicine's biggest challenge for the future.[8] Determining the quality of evidence requires not only an understanding of a particular

No funding was received for the preparation of this manuscript.
a University of Florida Health Science Center, Jacksonville, FL, USA
b Division of Orthopedic Trauma Surgery, University of Florida - Shands Jacksonville, 655 West 8th Street, ACC Building, 2nd Floor/Ortho, Jacksonville, FL 32209, USA
c Department of Health Services, University of Washington, Seattle, USA
d AO Foundation, Stettbachstrasse 6, 8600 Duebendorf, Switzerland
e Weill Cornell Medical College, New York, NY, USA
f Orthopedic Trauma Service, Hospital for Special Surgery, 535 East 70th Street, New York, NY 10021, USA
* Corresponding author. University of Florida - Shands Jacksonville, 655 West 8th Street, ACC Building, 2nd Floor/Ortho, Jacksonville, FL 32209.
E-mail address: Michael.suk@jax.ufl.edu

Orthop Clin N Am 41 (2010) 139–143
doi:10.1016/j.ocl.2009.11.002

study's materials, methods, and statistical analysis, but also the determinants of a patient's outcome. To do so, the outcomes instrument must be appropriately chosen and applied.

MEASURING OUTCOMES

Outcomes instruments that attempt to assess function and quality of life in orthopedic patients are multiplying. Today, there are nearly 400 general orthopedic musculoskeletal outcomes instruments being used for research or clinical purposes and more than 100 measures applicable to the spine alone.[9] Outcomes instruments can play an important role in the development of new procedures, techniques, and protocols in addition to providing some measure of quality. However, the musculoskeletal literature is filled with clinical justifications based on outcome results, such as "excellent," "good", or "poor" that can be at best, difficult to verify and at worst, misleading. Further, without a common language and standards, it is nearly impossible to adequately compare results against each other.

Taking into account the results of an appropriate outcomes measure is a critical step in recommending a course of treatment for musculoskeletal care. However, this can be a challenging task. In the process, one treatment protocol or intervention may be deemed better than another based on a specific desired end point (eg, range of motion), but not as good when based on another end point (eg, pain relief).

CLINICIAN-BASED OUTCOMES

One can think about outcome measures as being either clinician-based or patient-reported. Clinician-based outcomes are often physiologic and can be measured directly by the clinician. Examples include muscle strength, joint range of motion, gait abnormalities, limb length, and bony alignment. These physiologic measures, also known as "hard" or "objective" findings, are often used to infer a patient's functional ability. In contrast, patient-reported outcomes reflect a patient's perception of their functional ability, symptoms and quality of life. Because these are considered "soft" or "subjective," there has been some reluctance in the past to trust these types of outcomes measures.

A commonly held belief is that clinician-based outcomes are inherently objective. After all, clinicians measure directly a patient's motion, strength, or alignment. However, the key attribute to outcome objectivity is not dependent on who makes the assessment but rather on the reliability

or reproducibility of a finding.[10,11] There is substantial variability in many clinician-based outcomes. For example, interobserver agreement in determining motion of the spine[12,13] or extremities[14–17] is often poor. Muscle strength can be difficult to reproduce, particularly manually,[18] but also in some cases when a dynamometer is used.[19–21] Variability for simple imaging tests has also been documented.[22,23] On the other hand, reproducibility of many patient-reported outcomes can be quite high. By the standard of reliability, patient-reported outcomes can be as reliable as or more reliable than clinician-based outcomes, and therefore as or more objective.

Physicians have relied on clinician-based outcomes based on the belief that a strong link exists between those outcomes and patient well-being. However, such is often not the case.[24–27] For example, the severity of knee osteoarthritis is typically determined from orthogonal standing radiographs. Measurements of joint space compromise and alterations in the mechanical axis are assumed to correlate with a patient's overall quality of life. Yet, Bruyere and colleagues[28] showed that measurement of mean joint space width and the narrowest joint space point did not significantly correlate with pain, stiffness, or function derived from a patient-reported outcome measure, the Western Ontario and McMaster Osteoarthritis Index (WOMAC). In another example, 18 nonrheumatoid patients who underwent limited wrist fusion had poor wrist scores based on range of motion and grip strength that did not correlate highly with patient satisfaction or self-assessment of wrist performance.[29]

PATIENT-REPORTED OUTCOMES

It is increasingly recognized that traditional clinician-based outcome measures need to be complemented by measures that focus on the patient's concerns to evaluate interventions and identify whether one treatment is better than another.[30] Patient-reported outcomes are classified as either "general" or "disease-specific" measures of health-related quality of life. General measures are designed to be used across different diseases and across different demographic and cultural subgroups.[31] They are usually multidimensional and are designed to give a comprehensive and general overview of health-related quality of life. The most well known general measure of health-related quality of life is the Medical Outcomes Study Short Form-36, typically known as the SF-36.[32] General measures of health-related quality of life permit comparisons across populations with different health conditions and are more likely to detect unexpected effects of an intervention.[33] An important limitation of these measures is that they tend to be less responsive to changes in health status and are therefore less likely to detect the effects of a specific intervention compared with disease-specific measures of health-related quality of life.[34,35]

Musculoskeletal disease-specific measures of health-related quality of life, on the other hand, focus on aspects of health that are specific to an injury (eg, fracture), disease (eg, osteoarthritis), anatomic area (eg, knee), or population of interest (eg, athletes).[36] This specificity has been shown to contribute to a more responsive measure,[34,35] and is more able to detect smaller or important changes that occur over time in the particular disease studied.[31,37] For example, a hip-specific instrument designed for patients with osteoarthritis should be particularly responsive to important changes in patients receiving total hip arthroplasty because it focuses only on the most relevant items. Further assuming that the instrument has clear relevance to the patient's health problem, a disease-specific outcomes instrument will lead to greater patient acceptance, higher response rates, and improved data collection.[36] To ensure an adequate assessment of a patient's entire health-related quality of life, it is recommended that generic and disease-specific patient-reported outcomes measures be administered.[38,39]

EVALUATING EXISTING OUTCOMES MEASURES

Outcomes measures are designed to provide musculoskeletal clinicians and researchers the data necessary for self-improvement and critical evaluation. For the practicing clinician, evaluating the results of one's own intervention and assessing the results reported by others in the literature is often as important as understanding the technique itself. For epidemiologists and clinical researchers, outcomes measurements are essential for advancing education and developing new techniques. Questions one should consider when evaluating and choosing or developing the most appropriate outcome instruments for a given situation are listed in **Table 1**.

Consider the following hypothetical example: a clinical guideline is being proposed for the treatment of displaced distal radius fractures in the elderly population. In developing the guideline, surgical fixation and cast immobilization are being compared. Among the evidence being considered is a Level 1 study (assume this is a prospective, randomized clinical trial, with a 97% follow-up rate and a sample size exceeding 500 patients) in which the author has concluded, "cast immobilization is better than surgical fixation." As support for this conclusion, the author cites fewer complications (clinician-based outcome). At the same time, he notes a statistically significant lower union rate among the conservatively managed treatment group at 6 months (clinician-based outcome).

Assume at the 1-year follow-up, elderly patients suffering a distal radius fracture had statistically identical scores on the Patient Reported Wrist Evaluation (PRWE) in the surgical and conservatively managed groups (patient-reported outcome). The PRWE measures pain and function with a 0 to 100 point scale, and has been found to be valid, reliable, and responsive in several distal radius populations.[9]

So in considering the superiority of one method over another, this hypothetical example favored conservative management based on complication rates (a clinician-based outcome), surgical management if based on rate of nonunion (a clinician-based outcome), and no difference at 1 year based on a validated patient-reported outcome. This hypothetical example shows that the results and the ultimate clinical recommendation are highly dependent on the outcomes measured.

EVIDENCE-BASED ORTHOPEDICS: IS IT POSSIBLE?

Assessing success or failure based on the score itself can be misleading because of the variation

Table 1	
Questions to ask in evaluating an outcomes instrument	
1 Does the instrument measure the content you are interested in for your population?	✔
2 Does the measure produce a score that is interpretable? Does it make sense to you?	✔
3 Does the measure demonstrate reliability in a population you are interested in?	✔
4 Does the measure demonstrate validity in the population you are interested in?	✔
5 Does the measure demonstrate responsiveness in the patient population you are interested in?	✔
6 Will this measure be deemed acceptable by patients?	✔
7 Is this outcome feasible to administer clinically?	✔

in expectations of patients and surgeons. For example, consider the previous example. It is possible that an elderly patient operated on for a distal radius fracture, who scores 30 (lower the score the higher the function) on the PRWE, will have a better outcome than a young patient who scores 20. Although the scores may be contradictory, the patient with a PRWE score of 20 may actually have a poorer outcome because the patient considers the surgery a relative failure, even if the surgeon considers it a relative success. The opposite scenario could be said for the score of 30 on the PRWE resulting in a better outcome. Fundamentally, each patient has different expectations, and these expectations influence perceived outcomes.

Evidence-based medicine is founded on the "integration of clinical expertise with the best available clinical evidence and patients' values."[1] As we continue to explore its application to orthopedics, understanding the anatomy of outcomes measures and future directions in the integration of patient expectations will bring us to greater acceptance in clinical practice. The promise of evidence-based orthopedics is great and realization of that promise seems just on the horizon.

REFERENCES

1. Bourne RB, Maloney WJ, Wright JG. An AOA critical issue. The outcome of the outcomes movement. J Bone Joint Surg Am 2004;86:633–40.
2. Antes G, Galandi D, Bouillon B. What is evidence-based medicine? Langenbecks Arch Surg 1999; 384:409–16.
3. Bhandari M, Tornetta P III. Evidence-based orthopaedics: a paradigm shift. Clin Orthop Relat Res 2003;413:9–10.
4. McAlister FA, Graham I, Karr GW, et al. Evidence-based medicine and the practicing clinician. J Gen Intern Med 1999;14(2):36–42.
5. Henley MB, Turkelson C, Jacobs JJ, et al. AOA Symposium. Evidence-based medicine, the quality initiative and P4P: performance or paperwork? J Bone Joint Surg Am 2008;90:2781–90.
6. Bhandari M, Swiontkowski MF, Einhorn TA, et al. Interobserver agreement in the application of levels of evidence to scientific papers in the American volume of the journal of bone and joint surgery. J Bone Joint Surg Am 2002;84:1717–20.
7. Viveiros H, Mignott T, Bhandari M. Evidence-based orthopaedics: is it possible? J Long Term Eff Med Implants 2007;17(2):87–93.
8. Guyatt G, Cook D, Hayndes B. Evidence-based medicine has come a long way. BMJ 2004;329: m990–991.
9. Suk M, Hansen B, Norvell D, et al. AO handbook of musculoskeletal outcomes instruments and measures. 2nd edition. Basel (Switzerland): Thieme; 2009. February.
10. Feinstein AR. Clinical biostatistics. XLI. Hard science, soft data, and the challenges of choosing clinical variables in research. Clin Pharmacol Ther 1977;22:485–98.
11. Deyo RA. Using outcomes to improve quality of research and quality of care. J Am Board Fam Pract 1998;11:465–73.
12. Nelson MA, Allen P, Clamp SE, et al. Reliability and reproducibility of clinical findings in low-back pain. Spine 1979;4:97–101.
13. Miller SA, Mayer T, Cox R, et al. Reliability problems associated with the modified Schober technique for true lumbar flexion measurement. Spine 1992;17: 345–8.
14. Edwards TB, Bostick RD, Greene CC, et al. Interobserver and intraobserver reliability of the measurement of shoulder internal rotation by vertebral level. J Shoulder Elbow Surg 2002;11:40–2.
15. Hoving JL, Buchbinder R, Green S, et al. How reliably do rheumatologists measure shoulder movement? Ann Rheum Dis 2002;61:612–6.
16. Youdas JW, Bogard CL, Suman VJ. Reliability of goniometric measurements and visual estimates of ankle joint active range of motion obtained in a clinical setting. Arch Phys Med Rehabil 1993;74: 1113–8.
17. Bovens AM, van Baak MA, Vrencken JG, et al. Variability and reliability of joint measurements. Am J Sports Med 1990;18:58–63.
18. Hayes K, Walton JR, Szomor ZL, et al. Reliability of 3 methods for assessing shoulder strength. J Shoulder Elbow Surg 2002;11:33–9.
19. Moller M, Lind K, Styf J, et al. The reliability of isokinetic testing of the ankle joint and a heel-raise test for endurance. Knee Surg Sports Traumatol Arthrosc 2003;22:22.
20. Moreland J, Finch E, Stratford P, et al. Interrater reliability of six tests of trunk muscle function and endurance. J Orthop Sports Phys Ther 1997;26:200–8.
21. Agre JC, Magness JL, Hull SZ, et al. Strength testing with a portable dynamometer: reliability for upper and lower extremities. Arch Phys Med Rehabil 1987;68:454–8.
22. Koran LM. The reliability of clinical methods, data and judgments (second of two parts). N Engl J Med 1975;293:695–701.
23. Deyo RA, McNiesh LM, Cone RO 3rd. Observer variability in the interpretation of lumbar spine radiographs. Arthritis Rheum 1985;28:1066–70.
24. Torgerson WR, Dotter WE. Comparative roentgenographic study of the asymptomatic and symptomatic lumbar spine. J Bone Joint Surg Am 1976;58: 850–3.

25. Witt I, Vestergaard A, Rosenklint A. A comparative analysis of x-ray findings of the lumbar spine in patients with and without lumbar pain. Spine 1984; 9:298–300.

26. Wilson IB, Cleary PD. Linking clinical variables with health-related quality of life. A conceptual model of patient outcomes. JAMA 1995;273:59–65.

27. Khan AM, McLoughlin E, Giannakas K, et al. Hip osteoarthritis: where is the pain? Ann R Coll Surg Engl 2004;86:119–21.

28. Bruyere O, Honore A, Rovati LC, et al. Radiologic features poorly predict clinical outcomes in knee osteoarthritis. Scand J Rheumatol 2002;31:13–6.

29. Tomaino MM, Miller RJ, Burton RI. Outcome assessment following limited wrist fusion: objective wrist scoring versus patient satisfaction. Contemp Orthop 1994;28:403–10.

30. Slevin ML, Plant H, Lynch D, et al. Who should measure quality of life, the doctor or the patient? Br J Cancer 1988;57:109–12.

31. McSweeny AJ, Creer TL. Health-related quality-of-life assessment in medical care. Dis Mon 1995;41: 1–71.

32. Ware JE Jr, Sherbourne CD. The MOS 36-item short-form health survey (SF-36). I. Conceptual framework and item selection. Med Care 1992;30:473–83.

33. Kessler RC, Mroczek DK. Measuring the effects of medical interventions. Med Care 1995;33: AS109–19.

34. Guyatt GH, Feeny DH, Patrick DL. Measuring health-related quality of life. Ann Intern Med 1993; 118:622–9.

35. Wright JG, Young NL. A comparison of different indices of responsiveness. J Clin Epidemiol 1997;50:239–46.

36. Fitzpatrick R, Davey C, Buxton MJ, et al. Evaluating patient-based outcome measures for use in clinical trials. Health Technol Assess 1998;2:1–74.

37. Patrick DL, Deyo RA. Generic and disease-specific measures in assessing health status and quality of life. Med Care 1989;27:S217–32.

38. Fletcher A, Gore S, Jones D, et al. Quality of life measures in health care. II: design, analysis, and interpretation. BMJ 1992;305:1145–8.

39. Guyatt G, Feeny D, Patrick D. Issues in quality-of-life measurement in clinical trials. Control Clin Trials 1991;12:81S–90S.

Challenges of Randomized Controlled Surgical Trials

Angela J. Campbell, BS[a], Anita Bagley, MPH, PhD[b,c],
Ann Van Heest, MD[d], Michelle A. James, MD[a,c],*

KEYWORDS

- Randomized controlled trials • Surgery • Research
- Children • Evidence-based medicine

The concept of evidence-based medicine has gained broad support in the medical community, because clinical decisions based on information from rigorous scientific study are most likely to provide optimal care.[1]

When researchers attempt to answer clinical questions, they must first decide whether to observe the events taking place in the subjects (observational study) or to introduce an intervention and analyze its effects on the subjects (randomized controlled trial).[2] Observational studies such as Cohort studies (prospective or retrospective) and the cross-sectional study currently dominate the surgical literature.[3] These may be the best methods if researchers are studying the outcomes of uncommon treatments or diseases, if funding is scarce,[2] or if there is only 1 acceptable intervention and the physician is ethically obligated to offer it. However, observational studies can only demonstrate an association between observations, and therefore provide an inferior level of evidence to the other study designs, or a randomized controlled trial (RCT), which has the ability to show causality.[2] RCTs are ethically grounded in clinical equipoise. If one treatment has not been proven better than another, a state of clinical equipoise exists, and subjects can ethically be randomly assigned to an intervention to reduce the effects that could influence the outcome.[2] The results observed in such a study are more likely to be the consequence of the intervention.

RCTs may further reduce the potential for bias or other confounding factors due to chance by blinding. Blinded RCTs are the prevalent method used to compare pharmaceutical interventions, and theoretically, these would be the best way to compare different surgical procedures, and to compare surgery with nonoperative treatment options. Pharmaceutical trials can be designed such that subjects alone or subjects and researchers are blinded to the drug administered (single-blinded versus double-blinded studies). In double-blinded studies (the most stringent form of blinding) study participants, caregivers, and investigators do not know the treatment group that a subject has been assigned to until the study has ended. Thus, randomization prevents bias at

[a] Department of Orthopaedics, Shriners Hospitals for Children, Northern California, 2425 Stockton Boulevard, Sacramento, CA 95817, USA
[b] Motion Analysis Laboratory, Shriners Hospitals for Children, Northern California, 2425 Stockton Boulevard, Sacramento, CA 95817, USA
[c] Department of Orthopaedic Surgery, University of California, Davis School of Medicine, 4860 Y Street, Suite 3800, Sacramento, CA 95817, USA
[d] Department of Orthopaedic Surgery, University of Minnesota, 2450 Riverside Avenue South, Suite R200, Minneapolis, MN 55454, USA
* Corresponding author. Department of Orthopaedics, Shriners Hospitals for Children, Northern California, 2425 Stockton Boulevard, Sacramento, CA 95817.
E-mail address: mjames@shrinenet.org

Orthop Clin N Am 41 (2010) 145–155
doi:10.1016/j.ocl.2009.11.001

the time of allocation to a treatment group, and blinding prevents bias during the data collection process.[2]

Blinding in surgical trials is much more challenging than in pharmaceutical trials. The surgeon cannot be blinded to the procedure, so a double-blind design is not feasible. Blinding of patients is possible in a surgical trial if the subjects in one of the treatment arms receive a placebo or sham surgery, but there are practical and ethical barriers to this practice.

RCTs are the gold standard in study design and they play a vital role in increasing medical knowledge about treatment effectiveness and supporting clinical decisions with evidence-based data. However, surgical RCTs are not commonly performed and reported in the scientific literature in general,[1,4–9] and are even scarcer in orthopedic surgery, because of the many challenges described in this article.

This article discusses the barriers to implementation of surgical RCTs, using the authors' experience with a pediatric orthopedic RCT in which children are randomized to surgical versus nonsurgical treatment as a case study to illustrate some of the key points.

RCTS AND EVIDENCE-BASED MEDICINE

Because data produced from blinded RCTs allows researchers to draw conclusions about the cause and effect relationships of interventions and outcomes,[10] they have become known as the gold standard of evidence-based medicine.[6,11–13] The original definition of evidence-based medicine is "the conscientious, explicit, and judicious use of current best evidence in making decisions about the care of individual patients."[14] Randomization does not guarantee that every variable that could potentially bias the results is accounted for, but it does reduce or eliminate the selection bias of the researcher and the subject.[12] Because results of blinded RCTs have the lowest chance of bias, these are assumed to provide the best scientific evidence available. Study design rigor is rated using the Oxford Center for Evidence-Based Medicine Levels of Evidence, which are used or adapted for use by medical journals for published results.[15,16] According to this rating scheme, the blinded RCT provides the highest levels of evidence, Level 1 or Level 2 (**Table 1** for an adaptation of the Oxford Levels of Evidence used by the *Journal of Bone and Joint Surgery*).

New surgical procedures are developed by a single surgeon or a group of surgeons who perform a new procedure and observe the results in either a case series report or a retrospective or prospective cohort study.[6,17] Results from this level of evidence are potentially biased by patient selection and the surgeon's enthusiasm for the procedure, in addition to small study cohorts and problems with data collection and data analysis. Furthermore, this approach does not allow for controlled comparison between surgical procedures or comparison of surgical treatment with a nonsurgical intervention.[17]

Several barriers to achieving Level 1 evidence are inherent in the design of a surgical trial. Subject recruitment is difficult when the study design includes randomizing to surgery versus nonsurgical treatment arms,[6] because of perceived lack of clinical equipoise by the surgeon, and/or potential subject preference. Randomizing subjects to 1 of 2 surgical treatment arms may be more agreeable to potential subjects because both treatments still involve surgery. Blinding techniques are also difficult in surgical trials. The surgeon cannot be blinded to a subject's treatment arm, and unless a study uses a placebo or sham surgery, it is difficult to blind the patient.

Sham surgical trials that blind the patient to the procedure performed are uncommon,[18–22] but these trials have the potential to provide clinicians with definitive answers to surgical questions. One well-known orthopedic sham surgery study provided high-level evidence that arthroscopic surgery for arthritis of the knee was no more effective than the placebo or sham surgery.[21] However, the use of sham surgery raises ethical concerns,[9,17,19] as discussed later, because a subject undergoing sham surgery is exposed to the risks of surgery without the potential benefits.

BARRIERS TO PERFORMING AND PUBLISHING RCTS

There has been a recent increase in RCTs reported in the orthopedic literature. A review of 36,293 articles in orthopedic journals found 671 RCTs and 12 meta-analyses published between 1966 and 1999. Over 75% of the RCTs were published between 1990 and 1999 (528 RCTs), whereas only 122 RCTs were published between 1980 and 1989, and 21 RCTs were published between 1968 and 1979.[5]

Despite recent increases, only about 7% of articles in surgical journals are RCTs.[8] Another review found that only 3.4% of all articles in leading surgical journals were RCTs.[9] Of RCTs published in the same leading surgical journals during a 10-year period, less than half compared the results of surgery with a nonsurgical alternative treatment.[9] These deficiencies are well described,[3,5–7,23] and

Table 1
Levels of evidence for primary research question

	Types of Studies		
	Therapeutic Studies Investigating the Results of Treatment	**Prognostic Studies Investigating the Effect of a Patient Characteristic on the Outcome of Disease**	**Diagnostic Studies Investigating a Diagnostic Test**
Level 1	• High-quality RCT with statistically significant difference or no statistically significant difference but narrow confidence intervals[a] • Systematic review[b] of Level 1 RCTs (and study results were homogeneous[c])	• High-quality prospective study[d] (all patients were enrolled at the same point in their disease with ≥80% follow-up of enrolled patients) • Systematic review[b] of Level 1 studies	• Testing of previously developed diagnostic criteria in series of consecutive patients (with universally applied reference gold standard) • Systematic review[b] of Level 1 studies
Level 2	• Lesser-quality RCT (eg, <80% follow-up, no blinding, or improper randomization) • Prospective[d] comparative study[e] • Systematic review[b] of Level 2 studies or Level 1 studies with inconsistent results	• Retrospective[f] study • Untreated controls from an RCT • Lesser-quality prospective study (eg, patients enrolled at different points in their disease or <80% follow-up) • Systematic review[b] of Level 2 studies	• Development of diagnostic criteria on the basis of consecutive patients (with universally applied reference gold standard) • Systematic review[b] of Level 2 studies
Level 3	• Case-control study[g] • Retrospective[f] comparative study[e] • Systematic review[b] of Level 3 studies	• Case-control study[g]	• Study of nonconsecutive patients (without consistently applied reference gold standard) • Systematic review[b] of Level 3 studies
Level 4	• Case series[h]		• Case-control study • Poor reference standard
Level 5	• Expert opinion	• Expert opinion	• Expert opinion

[a] A complete assessment of the quality of individual studies requires critical appraisal of all aspects of the study design.
[b] A combination of results from two or more previous studies.
[c] Studies provided consistent results.
[d] Study was started before the first patient enrolled.
[e] Patients treated one way (eg, with cemented hip arthroplasty) compared with patients treated another way (eg, with cementless hip arthroplasty) at the same institution.
[f] Study was started after the first patient enrolled.
[g] Patients identified for the study on the basis of their outcome (eg, failed total hip arthroplasty), called "cases," are compared with those who did not have the outcome (eg, had a successful total hip arthroplasty), called "controls."
[h] Patients treated one way with no comparison group of patients treated another way.

Adapted from material published by the Center for Evidence-Based Medicine, Oxford, UK. For more information, please see http://www.cebm.net. *Source:* Levels of evidence for primary research question. August 25, 2009. Available at: http://www2.ejbjs.org/misc/instrux.dtl#23levels [last accessed September 29, 2009]; with permission.

the surgical literature lags behind other medical specialties in these respects.[24,25]

Specialty surgical literature does not contain many RCTs. A search of the *Journal of Hand Surgery* (American) from 1976 to 1994 (volumes 1–19) found that only 1% of all the published articles were RCTs.[8] A search of all English-language literature for clinical trials in pediatric surgery from 1966 to 1999 identified only 134 RCTs out of 80,377 articles (0.17%).[6] These RCTs studied analgesia (49%), antibiotics (13%), extra-corporeal membrane oxygenation (7%), and treatment of gastrointestinal conditions, burns, congenital anomalies, trauma and cancer, minimally invasive surgery, and vascular access (each less than 5%).[6] Furthermore, of these 134 RCTs, 81% (109 studies) compared 2 medical therapies in surgical patients, 12% (16 studies) compared 2 surgical treatments, and 7% (9 studies) compared medical versus surgical treatment.[6]

Surgical RCTs are uncommon for several reasons, including ethical issues, patient and surgeon preferences, irreversibility of surgical treatment, expense and follow-up time, and difficulties associated with randomization and blinding.[8] Barriers to conducting successful RCTs also include the relative infrequency of the disease state under consideration, lack of community equipoise regarding standards of care, limited availability of diagnostic tools, and the challenges of enrolling children in RCTs.[6,26] Uncommon diseases cannot be studied at a single center, but multicenter trials are expensive and complicated to conduct.[6] Although nonoperative interventions are more common in pediatric orthopedics than in other orthopedic subspecialties, studies of pediatric surgical interventions comparing the results of surgery with nonsurgical interventions are especially uncommon.

Clinical equipoise, or genuine uncertainty about the best treatment, is a necessary criteria for randomizing subjects to treatment. Because of the deficit of RCTs, surgeons tend to rely on anecdotal data for making treatment decisions, thus creating a bias against the presumption of clinical equipoise. The data from biased studies may prematurely eliminate or falsely alter assumptions of clinical equipoise, interfering with the conduction of more scientifically rigorous research.[6]

QUALITY OF PUBLISHED RCTS

The actual level of evidence provided by an RCT depends on the quality of the study design, including the methodology of randomization and blinding, and on the rigor of the analysis and interpretation of results.[15] It is possible to conduct a poor-quality RCT that may be just as biased if randomization and blinding never occurred; in fact, the quality of some of the few surgical RCTs that have reached publication appears to be poor. Reviews and meta-analyses have revealed major flaws in methodology and study design.[4,6,7,13,23,25–29]

Several different assessment tools can be used to evaluate the quality of RCTs. The most commonly used tools are the Chalmers index and the Jadad score.[26] These tools are not entirely applicable to surgical RCTs because of the weight they give to blinding techniques. For example, the Jadad score was originally validated for RCTs assessing treatment of pain.[29] Surgical trials automatically score poorly on these scales because of the inherent design limitations, which include the impossibility of blinding the surgeon to the treatment and the rarity of blinding the subject in a sham surgical trial.

Another assessment tool, the Detsky scale, helps evaluate the quality of RCTs but does not penalize surgical trials for their inability to blind participants and researchers.[26] However, a Canadian study found that even using the Detsky scale only 19% of all pediatric orthopedic RCTs published in 5 well-recognized journals between 1995 and 2005 met the satisfactory level of methodological quality.[26] A separate study that also used the Detsky scale to assess the quality of RCTs in the *Journal of Bone and Joint Surgery* from 1988 to 2000 found that only 40% of the studies met the standard of acceptability.[7,26] Surgical trials received slightly lower quality scores than did drug trials (63.9% compared with 72.8% according to Detsky score standardization).[7] This study also found that funding of a trial and involvement of at least 1 epidemiologist were associated with better RCT quality.[7] Lack of funding may play a significant role in the quality of surgical RCTs,[9] because surgical RCTs lag significantly behind drug trials in terms of funding from the National Institutes of Health. Surgical trials are less likely to be funded than nonsurgical trials, and awards for surgical grants average 5% to 27% less than nonsurgical grants.[30] In the same study that identified 134 pediatric surgical RCTs over a 33-year period, only 13% cited a biostatistician as an author or a consultant, 7% stated that they received funding from either National Institutes of Health or Medical Research Council, and 65% mentioned no funding source at all.[6]

The most common methodological flaw in pediatric surgical trials is failure to identify specific inclusion and exclusion criteria, and failure to describe eligible patients who choose not to participate.[6] The majority of studies that tracked patient withdrawal excluded the data from these patients from statistical analysis. In addition, many RCTs state that the trial was randomized and blinded or double-blinded, but do not discuss the method of randomization or blinding.[23,31] RCTs using flawed methods of randomization overstate the effect of intervention.[23,32] In an observational study that analyzed the quality of allocation concealment in 250 RCTs from 33 meta-analyses (from the Cochrane Pregnancy and Childbirth Database), trials that had inadequate concealment techniques exaggerated treatment effect by 41%. Trials that had unclear concealment techniques exaggerated treatment effect by 30%.[33]

Additional problems with methodology include failure to perform a power analysis, in which the researchers identify the primary outcome measure before performing the study.[23,31] This is necessary to determine the power of the study, or whether sample sizes are adequate to detect clinical differences. An analysis of 760 abstracts accepted for presentation at the British Association of Pediatric Surgeons Annual Congress during a 5-year period (1996–2000) revealed that 9 were RCTs. A review of these 9 trials revealed that the actual number of subjects enrolled was far below what was needed to find a significant difference between treatment arms, raising the likelihood of type 2 errors (an incorrect conclusion of no difference between treatment arms when a difference does exist).[23] Underpowered studies such as these may lead to an incorrect interpretation of the data when a clinically important difference might exist.[23]

POTENTIAL SUBJECTS' LACK OF COMPREHENSION AND SUPPORT OF RANDOMIZATION AS A BARRIER TO RECRUITMENT

Appropriate study design, data collection, and analysis can solve many of the problems associated with RCTs, but subject recruitment remains a challenge. Potential subjects may not understand the concept of randomization and what it means to them if they choose to participate in an RCT. Twenty subjects participating in an RCT that randomized them to 1 of 3 different treatment arms for benign prostatic disease (laser therapy, standard surgery, or conservative management) were interviewed to gain a qualitative assessment of their understanding of randomization.[34] Most participants (14 out of 20) could describe certain aspects of randomization, such as involvement of chance, but their understanding of key terms used by the researchers, such as random and trial,

differed from the researchers' intent. To study participants, random meant that treatments were allocated without purpose or control, whereas trial meant that something was being tested. For instance, patients interpreted their participation in a clinical trial as testing new therapies or technologies. They could understand that the laser therapy was on trial, or being tested, because it was a new technology, but they did not comprehend that the standard surgical treatment was also on trial. In addition, it was difficult for them to comprehend that the clinician was not going to assign them to a treatment arm based on their individual characteristics, such as specific symptoms, clinical findings, or age. They believed that their doctors would decide the best treatment for them using information from their medical record.[34]

An additional study looked at 3 ideas behind the concept of randomization: whether the public could accept that the doctor did not know which of the 2 treatments was better (clinical equipoise); that in situations where the best treatment is unknown, it is acceptable to assign treatment randomly; and that there are scientific benefits to randomly assigning treatments in an RCT.[35] A total of 344 participants were asked about scenarios that involved uncertainty in clinical, research, and other nonmedical contexts. About half of the participants could not accept that a clinician could be completely uncertain about a treatment, and they were less comfortable with uncertainty in clinical situations than nonmedical contexts. Most participants found it unacceptable to assign a treatment at random. Participants also did not recognize that random treatment assignment was a way to understand and compare treatment effects. Some participants made false assumptions to justify randomization, concluding that it removes the responsibility of making difficult decisions from doctors or parents, or that it gives the hospital a way to ration an expensive treatment. It seems that potential study subjects do not recognize, or are not willing to accept the idea that clinicians may not know the best treatment for an individual. When they give consent to become subjects and participate in research, patients assume that the treatment that they receive is selected for them by their doctor because it is best for them, even though they are told this will not be the case in an RCT.[35]

Although most people do seem to understand the concept of randomization involving elements of chance, such as someone having an equal chance of being assigned to one option as another, most people do not find it acceptable to use randomization for research on clinical treatment.[36] In a study that examined the layperson's ability to understand and accept the concept of randomization in a clinical trial context, of the randomization methods correctly identified by participants, few were acceptable to them in a clinical trial scenario. The acceptability of one randomization method was increased by including a scientific justification (randomization by computer), although acceptability of this method still remained low.[36] This study also indicated that researchers tend to discuss only those parts of the study that are easy for the patients to understand instead of the parts that might be more difficult,[36] raising important concerns about the specific process that occurs when a researcher obtains informed consent for an RCT. It is also possible that parents are more reluctant to give permission for their children to receive a random treatment assignment than they might be for themselves. Potential participants may need more information about study design than they typically receive, especially for studies involving children. More accessible written information or follow-up telephone conversations with a researcher might help with misunderstandings of random allocation in RCTs.[35]

OTHER BARRIERS TO SUBJECT RECRUITMENT AND RETENTION

Many RCTs overestimate the ability to recruit subjects and recruit less than 75% of the total projected. It has been estimated that a maximum of 60% of eligible patients will agree to participate in an RCT and of those enrolled, up to 50% will drop out of the trial.[8] Documented reasons for withdrawal of subjects from recent studies include lengthy study visits or not having time for the study (47.1%), moved out of town (23.5%), and committed to other research (17.6%).[37] Recruitment strategies to improve subject enrollment include[1] provision of information before invitation to join study (prewarning),[2] provision of extra information about study benefits and risks,[3] changes to the study design to account for patient preference including not having a placebo study arm,[4] changes to the consent process such as increased time for discussion and education,[5] and incentives.[38,39]

Because dropouts threaten the validity of the research findings, researchers have conducted a review of studies with a primary focus on strategies to retain participants. Studies with lower retention rates (<86%) have reported the use of fewer retention strategies than those with higher retention rates.[38] Multiple strategies should be adopted to improve retention and minimize

participant burden, including systematic methods for patient contact, scheduling appointments and monitoring attendance, updating contact information every 2 months, and making multiple attempts to contact subjects to obtain complete data. Strategies to minimize participant burden include conducting interviews at home and providing refreshments in the follow-up clinic.[38,39]

Retention of pediatric participants depends on parent and child behavior. In a study of interventions to improve adherence to a diabetes treatment regimen, demographic patterns could predict whether a patient would complete the study. For children, these factors included age, sex, health status, and cognitive, emotional, and behavioral functioning. For adults, factors included age, education, and psychological functioning. Patients who completed the study on time were more likely to have private medical insurance and parents with some college education; those who completed the study later than expected were more likely to be boys and to have parents with mild depression; and those who withdrew from the study were more likely to report poor quality of life and were more likely to have parents who did not work outside the home.[37] Handpicking potential study participants for demographic criteria associated with better participation might improve retention, but would clearly introduce selection bias and ethical concerns.

Strategies to improve recruitment and retention for pediatric participants include study visits that coincide with clinic visits, providing children with small toys for participating, and providing rewards for completing telephone interviews. The best study design has interventions at regular clinic visits that can be completed within 1 year. This reduces withdrawal rates to about 10%, making recruitment less burdensome for the researchers and enhancing the validity of the study findings.[37]

ALTERNATIVES TO SURGICAL RCTS

Because of the challenges faced by researchers when attempting to perform research on surgical treatment that will provide a high level of evidence, alternative methodologies to RCTs have been described.

The expertise-based surgical RCT helps to eliminate differences between surgeons performing the surgical technique in question.[8] Because surgical procedures have a significant learning curve before a level of expertise is reached, this trial design ensures that all study participants assigned to a particular technique by randomization are also assigned to a surgeon who is an expert in that technique. This is done because surgeons who are most familiar with a technique are presumed to have the best outcomes.[8] Using surgeons who are considered experts in a specific surgical technique helps eliminate expertise bias and maintains community equipoise.[8]

The randomized consent design RCT is a useful design for surgeons who prefer to tell their patients with certainty which treatment they will receive.[11] In this RCT design, a patient is randomized to a treatment arm first and is then asked for informed consent after the physician explains which treatment has been selected for them.[11] This may help alleviate some of the mistrust that may occur between doctor and patient when trying to explain that their treatment will be chosen at random.

Another alternative is the patient preference design RCT, which allows patients who have a clear preference for a treatment arm to still be enrolled in the research study.[11] The physician presents all treatment arms to the patient and the patient is able to decide which one they prefer. Patients who do not have a preference are randomized. Proponents of the patient preference design argue that the classic RCT does not truly represent the true clinic setting where patient and physician have free choice. In addition, patients who choose a particular treatment arm are more likely to represent the population of those most likely to choose that treatment in the future.[11]

All of these alternatives are less rigorous than RCTs, because in the process of modifying the randomization process, they weaken the ability of this process to reduce bias.

ETHICAL CONCERNS REGARDING SURGICAL RCTS

Conducting RCTs to answer pediatric surgical questions is a unique challenge, particularly when recruiting children as participants and when types of treatment are different. Even if recruitment barriers are surmounted, ethical concerns remain.

It is unethical to conduct an RCT on a surgical intervention that has already been widely accepted[8] and proven superior. If one treatment is better than another, the surgeon is ethically bound to treat the patient with the better treatment, and the clinical equipoise required for randomization does not exist.[40] However, if the evidence in support of 2 alternative treatments is limited, neither is clearly superior, and both have supporters, even though an individual surgeon may have a preference for a particular treatment, community equipoise can exist.[11,41] The ethics of randomization when 1 of the

treatment options is surgery have been questioned.[24] However, if true community equipoise exists and informed consent is properly obtained, an RCT comparing surgery to nonsurgical treatment can be ethical.[8,11] There are several examples of RCTs that have successfully compared medical and surgical therapies and have addressed these ethical concerns.[24,42,43]

Another argument against RCTs is that randomization detracts from the quality of care received by the patient because the process of randomization threatens the physician-patient relationship.[11,40] This position is difficult to refute as there is no standardized method of measuring the quality of the physician-patient relationship.

The greatest methodological challenge for surgical RCTs is the blinding of participants. As previously mentioned, 1 method of blinding surgical trials is the use of placebo or sham surgery. This approach engenders significant ethical issues. Performing the incision without the intervention is controversial.[9,17] Sham surgery exposes the patient to the risks of anesthesia and surgery, including infection and pain, without the potential benefits of the surgical intervention.[17] Furthermore, once the sham operation has been performed, the patient must be deceived at all subsequent follow-ups with medical providers in order for them to be truly blinded to their treatment arm.[17]

A few sham surgical trials have been reported in the orthopedic literature. In 2002, a study by Moseley and colleagues[21] evaluated the effectiveness of arthroscopic surgery for arthritis of the knee. One treatment group underwent a full arthroscopic debridement, 1 underwent arthroscopic lavage with irrigation fluid alone, and the last group received three 1-cm incisions with no other surgical intervention. This study found that arthroscopic surgery for advanced arthritis was no more effective than the sham operation.[17] As is inherent in research, the benefits of this study accrued to future patients (who were spared an ineffective treatment), not to the subjects who accrued the risks. Some have argued that sham surgeries should be viewed the same way as additional blood draws, radiographs, lumbar punctures, and biopsies, and that study participants randomized to a sham surgery receive many benefits, including pain medicine, frequent follow-up, exercise programs, counseling, and the placebo effect of surgery.[17]

If sham surgery is not a suitable methodology, blinding can be limited to the outcome assessor. In this modification, the surgeon and patient are not blinded, but the person assessing the results does not know the treatment. If the study

Table 2
UECP RCT study design

	Surgery	Botox	Therapy
Treatment	First evaluation		
	FCU to ECRB, PT release, adductor release, EPL re-routing	1st injection (to FCU, PT, adductor)	Regular ongoing treatment
Splinting and therapy	8 sessions supervised OT followed by home therapy program	8 sessions supervised OT followed by home therapy program	8 sessions supervised OT followed by home therapy program
3 months	N/A	2nd injection	N/A
6 months	Second evaluation		
	N/A	3rd injection	N/A
12 months	Third evaluation		

Abbreviations: ECRB, extensor carpi radialis brevis; EPL, extensor pollicis longus; FCU, flexor carpi ulnaris; OT, operating theatre; PT, physical therapy.

Data from Shriners Hospitals for Children Northern California. Multi-center study: comparison of functional outcomes of tendon transfer surgery, botulinum toxin injections and regular on-going treatment in hemiplegic upper extremity cerebral palsy (UECP). Shriners Hospitals for Children Clinical Grant #9196, 2005.

compares 2 operations with different incisions, or surgical and nonsurgical treatment, the affected extremity can be covered during outcome assessment so that the assessor cannot identify the intervention.

However, as a result of using less rigorous methodologies than sham surgery, numerous surgical interventions have become routine based on unreliable evidence of patient outcomes.[17] Because the sham surgery methodology always engenders

Table 3
Shriners Hospitals UECP participant enrollment log

Site	Approached	Refused	Enrolled	Dropped Out	Refusal Numbers	Reasons for Refusals
1	22	15	7		6	Did not want randomization
					2	Request surgery only
					2	Request therapy only
					1	Request botox only
					3	Reason unknown
					1	No intervention wanted at this time
2	8	3	5		2	Did not want randomization
					1	Request surgery only
3	0	0	0		N/A	
4	1	0	0		N/A	
5	11	6	5	2	3	Request surgery only
					2	Did not want surgery
					1	Not interested
6	10	5	5	1	5	Request surgery only
7	3	0	3		N/A	
8	10	8	2		2	Did not want randomization
					3	Request surgery only
					2	Request botox only
					1	Reason unknown
Total	65	37	27	3	37	

Data from Shriners Hospitals for Children Clinical.

the ethical concerns of subjecting subjects to substantial risks with no potential for benefit and because of the need for ongoing deception of subjects, only studies that are well designed and likely to answer extremely pertinent surgical questions should consider sham surgery as a methodology, and as for all human research, the scrutiny and approval of the Human Subjects Committee is imperative.

CASE STUDY

Shriners Hospitals for Children Northern California is the leading site for a multicenter study comparing functional outcomes of 3 different treatment algorithms: (1) tendon transfer surgery, (2) botulinum toxin injections, and (3) regular ongoing treatment (therapy) for hemiplegic upper extremity cerebral palsy (UECP) since 2004. Although Shriners Hospitals treat thousands of children disabled by UECP, the optimal treatment for this condition is unknown. Typically, treatment for children with UECP focuses on balancing spastic muscles to improve joint position and function and prevent fixed deformities by using any of these 3 treatment modalities: therapeutic stretching and splinting, botulinum toxin injections, and/or surgical intervention (muscle release and transfer).

Because none of these 3 treatment methods (therapy, botulinum toxin, or surgery) is known to be superior, clinical equipoise exists regarding the best treatment for children with UECP. This study was designed as an RCT to compare satisfaction, function, and quality of life outcomes of these 3 treatment methods, to provide the highest level of evidence possible. Inclusion and exclusion criteria were established and agreed on by all participating centers. To be included in the study, all potential subjects must be candidates for the muscle release and tendon transfer surgery. **Table 2** shows a summary of the UECP study protocol. The therapy group serves as the control group. Subjects randomized to this group receive only regular, ongoing treatment according to a standardized protocol of stretching and splinting that is also administered to the botulinum toxin injection and surgery groups. Physicians, subjects, and treating therapists are not blinded, but functional evaluations are videotaped with the affected forearm, wrist, palm, and thumb covered by stockingette and a bandaid, and the therapist rating the videotaped functional evaluations is blinded to the treatment arm. A power analysis based on the most well-validated function test indicated that 48 subjects were needed.

Table 4
Reasons for refusal totals

Refusals	Reason
10	Did not want randomization
14	Request surgery only
2	Request therapy only
3	Request botox only
1	No intervention wanted at this time
4	Reason unknown
1	Not interested
2	Did not want surgery
37	Total

This study has encountered some of the challenges previously reported for RCTs that compare surgery with nonsurgical treatment,[6] especially limited recruitment. Because this was anticipated, several measures were taken to maximize recruitment. Participation may be enhanced by the fact that after 1 year of study participation, parents and patients can choose to receive their treatment of choice. Delaying these treatment options for a year does not present any known disadvantage. Researchers also thought that the reversibility of botulinum toxin injections would allow randomization to this treatment arm seem more advantageous. To boost retention, the study was designed to last for only 1 year, with visits coinciding with clinic appointments. Study participants and their families were given a printed schedule of their treatment and evaluation appointments, reminder calls are placed before each visit, and contact information is verified at each visit.

Although these precautions have successfully maximized retention (3 of 27 subjects [11%] have dropped out), recruitment rates have varied widely between 9 participating sites, from 0 to 100%, with 37 of 65 potential subjects declining to participate (65% refusal rate) (**Table 3**). Reasons for refusal also vary between sites and include specific requests for one treatment arm over another (14 of 37 wanted surgery) or because parents did not want to randomize their child to treatment (10 of 37) (**Table 4**).

SUMMARY

Blinded RCTs for pharmaceutical trials are considered the gold standard of evidence-based medicine because they can determine causality between an intervention and an outcome. Although blinded RCTs have been accepted as the best evidence-based method for pharmaceutical and other nonsurgical research questions, adoption of blinded RCTs to answer surgical questions has been slow,[24,25] especially for studies involving pediatric patients. As discussed, many questions about surgical treatment cannot be answered by a blinded RCT, and for questions that can be answered using this methodology, recruitment for surgical RCTs is challenging, as exemplified by our case study. Alternatives to the traditional RCT have been suggested to attempt to circumvent the problems encountered in performing surgical RCTs,[8,11,40,44] but these have ethical, scientific, and statistical drawbacks,[11] and the traditional blinded RCT remains the most scientifically rigorous method for answering important surgical questions.

However, even the traditional RCT is still only our best attempt to obtain a representative sample population that is a "statistical abstraction of the truth."[11] The blinded RCT remains the gold standard of trial design, but an RCT can result in erroneous conclusions.[40] Surgeons should not assume that studies labeled as Level 1 RCTs are necessarily high-quality studies, or that Level 1 studies always provide more reliable information than Level 2 studies. The value of blinded RCT findings is dependent on following strict guidelines for design, conduct, analysis, reporting, proper inclusion and exclusion criteria, power analysis to avoid underpowering the question, and satisfactory reporting of patient retention,[4,15] When deciding whether the results of an RCT warrant a change in their practice, surgeons should review the quality and the level of evidence a study provides.[4] Although non-randomized studies do not control for as many potential biases as RCTs, the information provided by these studies is often the best available, and therefore the basis for evidence-based clinical decisions.[11,12]

Investigators should first formulate a worthwhile answerable question. Then the surgical trials they develop should use the highest quality and most appropriate study design possible to either definitively answer the question at hand, or to provide information that will allow future investigators to shed more light on the topic with subsequent meta-analysis.[7]

REFERENCES

1. Hardin WD Jr, Stylianos S, Lally KP. Evidence-based practice in pediatric surgery. J Pediatr Surg 1999; 34(5):908–12 [discussion: 912–3].

2. Hulley SB, Cummings SR, Browner WS, et al, editors. Designing clinical research. 3rd edition. Philadelphia: Wolters Kluwer Health; 2007. p. 367.

3. Devereaux PJ, McKee MD, Yusuf S. Methodologic issues in randomized controlled trials of surgical interventions. Clin Orthop Relat Res 2003;413: 25–32.

4. Poolman RW, Struijs PA, Krips R, et al. Does a "Level I evidence" rating imply high quality of reporting in orthopaedic randomised controlled trials? BMC Med Res Methodol 2006;6:44.

5. Kiter E, Karatosun V, Gunal I. Do orthopaedic journals provide high-quality evidence for clinical practice? Arch Orthop Trauma Surg 2003;123(2–3):82–5.

6. Moss RL, Henry MC, Dimmitt RA, et al. The role of prospective randomized clinical trials in pediatric surgery: state of the art? J Pediatr Surg 2001; 36(8):1182–6.

7. Bhandari M, Richards RR, Sprague S, et al. The quality of reporting of randomized trials in the Journal of Bone and Joint Surgery from 1988 through 2000. J Bone Joint Surg Am 2002;84(3):388–96.

8. Chung KC, Burns PB. A guide to planning and executing a surgical randomized controlled trial. J Hand Surg Am 2008;33(3):407–12.

9. Cook JA. The challenges faced in the design, conduct and analysis of surgical randomised controlled trials. Trial 2009;10:9.

10. Rosner A. Fables or foibles: inherent problems with RCTs. J Manipulative Physiol Ther 2003;26(7):460–7.

11. Fung EK, Lore JM Jr. Randomized controlled trials for evaluating surgical questions. Arch Otolaryngol Head Neck Surg 2002;128(6):631–4.

12. Stel VS, Jager KJ, Zoccali C, et al. The randomized clinical trial: an unbeatable standard in clinical research? Kidney Int 2007;72(5):539–42.

13. Jacquier I, Boutron I, Moher D, et al. The reporting of randomized clinical trials using a surgical intervention is in need of immediate improvement: a systematic review. Ann Surg 2006;244(5):677–83.

14. Sackett DL, Rosenberg WM, Gray JA, et al. Evidence based medicine: what it is and what it isn't. BMJ 1996;312(7023):71–2.

15. Soucacos PN, Johnson EO, Babis G. Randomised controlled trials in orthopaedic surgery and traumatology: overview of parameters and pitfalls. Injury 2008;39(6):636–42.

16. Patel A, Wilke HJ 2nd, Mingay D, et al. Patient attitudes toward granting consent to participate in perioperative randomized clinical trials. J Clin Anesth 2004;16(6):426–34.

17. Wolf BR, Buckwalter JA. Randomized surgical trials and "sham" surgery: relevance to modern orthopaedics and minimally invasive surgery. Iowa Orthop J 2006;26:107–11.

18. Clark CC. The physician's role, "sham surgery," and trust: a conflict of duties? Am J Bioeth 2003;3(4):57–8.

19. Kirkley A, et al. A randomized trial of arthroscopic surgery for osteoarthritis of the knee. N Engl J Med 2008;359(11):1097–107.

20. Cobb LA, et al. An evaluation of internal-mammary-artery ligation by a double-blind technic. N Engl J Med 1959;260(22):1115–8.

21. Moseley JB, et al. A controlled trial of arthroscopic surgery for osteoarthritis of the knee. N Engl J Med 2002;347(2):81–8.

22. Beecher HK. Surgery as placebo. A quantitative study of bias. JAMA 1961;176:1102–7.

23. Curry JI, Reeves B, Stringer MD. Randomized controlled trials in pediatric surgery: could we do better? J Pediatr Surg 2003;38(4):556–9.

24. McLeod RS. Issues in surgical randomized controlled trials. World J Surg 1999;23(12):1210–4.

25. Trippel SB, et al. Symposium. How to participate in orthopaedic randomized clinical trials. J Bone Joint Surg Am 2007;89(8):1856–64.

26. Dulai SK, et al. A quality assessment of randomized clinical trials in pediatric orthopaedics. J Pediatr Orthop 2007;27(5):573–81.

27. Balasubramanian SP, et al. Standards of reporting of randomized controlled trials in general surgery: can we do better? Ann Surg 2006;244(5):663–7.

28. Chan S, Bhandari M. The quality of reporting of orthopaedic randomized trials with use of a checklist for nonpharmacological therapies. J Bone Joint Surg Am 2007;89(9):1970–8.

29. Gummesson C, Atroshi I, Ekdahl C. The quality of reporting and outcome measures in randomized clinical trials related to upper-extremity disorders. J Hand Surg Am 2004;29(4):727–34 [discussion: 735–7].

30. Rangel SJ, Efron B, Moss RL. Recent trends in National Institutes of Health funding of surgical research. Ann Surg 2002;236(3):277–86 [discussion: 286–7].

31. Li P, et al. Randomization and concealment in surgical trials: a comparison between orthopaedic and non-orthopaedic randomized trials. Arch Orthop Trauma Surg 2005;125(1):70–2.

32. Kunz R, Vist G, Oxman AD. Randomisation to protect against selection bias in healthcare trials. Cochrane Database Syst Rev 2007;(2): MR000012.

33. Schulz KF, et al. Empirical evidence of bias. Dimensions of methodological quality associated with estimates of treatment effects in controlled trials. JAMA 1995;273(5):408–12.

34. Featherstone K, Donovan JL. Random allocation or allocation at random? Patients' perspectives of participation in a randomised controlled trial. BMJ 1998;317(7167):1177–80.

35. Robinson EJ, et al. Lay conceptions of the ethical and scientific justifications for random allocation in clinical trials. Soc Sci Med 2004;58(4):811–24.

36. Kerr C, et al. Randomisation in trials: do potential trial participants understand it and find it acceptable? J Med Ethics 2004;30(1):80–4.

37. Driscoll KA, et al. Predictors of study completion and withdrawal in a randomized clinical trial of a pediatric diabetes adherence intervention. Contemp Clin Trials 2009.

38. Robinson KA, et al. Systematic review identifies number of strategies important for retaining study participants. J Clin Epidemiol 2007;60(8):757–65.

39. Mapstone J, Elbourne D, Roberts I. Strategies to improve recruitment to research studies. Cochrane Database Syst Rev 2007;(2):MR000013.

40. Rudicel S, Esdaile J. The randomized clinical trial in orthopaedics: obligation or option? J Bone Joint Surg Am 1985;67(8):1284–93.

41. Freedman B. Equipoise and the ethics of clinical research. N Engl J Med 1987;317(3):141–5.

42. Kerkhoffs GM, et al. Surgical versus conservative treatment for acute injuries of the lateral ligament complex of the ankle in adults. Cochrane Database Syst Rev 2007;(2):CD000380.

43. Handoll HH, Parker MJ. Conservative versus operative treatment for hip fractures in adults. Cochrane Database Syst Rev 2008;(3):CD000337.

44. Grundy DJ, Silver JR. Problems in the management of combined brachial plexus and spinal cord injuries. Int Rehabil Med 1981;3:57.

Optimal Treatment of Femoral Neck Fractures According to Patient's Physiologic Age: An Evidence-Based Review

Jason A. Lowe, MD[a], Brett D. Crist, MD[b],
Mohit Bhandari, MD, MSc, FRCSC[c], Tania A. Ferguson, MD[a],*

KEYWORDS
• Femoral neck fracture • Arthroplasty
• Narrative-review • Open reduction and internal fixation

For decades, the basic tenets of managing displaced femoral neck fractures have not changed, but the optimal treatment choice continues to be highly debated. The first step in management includes an assessment of the patient's physiologic age.[1] Chronologic age becomes less important in patients who are active with high functional demands, good bone quality, and few medical comorbidities. These patients are considered "young," whereas patients with poor bone quality and significant medical comorbidities are often considered "old" despite chronologic age.[2] The contemporary controversies associated with the treatment principles of displaced femoral neck fractures are distinct between these 2 age groups and will be considered individually in this review of the current evidence.

FEMORAL NECK FRACTURES IN YOUNG PATIENTS

Femoral neck fractures in physiologically young patients are managed differently than those in the elderly. These patients have fewer medical problems, sustain different fracture patterns, and have good bone quality. These patients typically have high functional demands and are not considered good candidates for hip replacement. Surgical timing, the role of capsulotomy, and the choice of internal fixation remain controversial.

Does Surgical Timing Matter?

Avascular necrosis
The most common justification for emergent care of femoral neck fractures in "young" patients has been to rapidly reestablish the blood supply to the femoral head and thus minimize the risk of avascular necrosis (AVN). Swiontkowski and colleagues[3] reported low rates of AVN (20%) in 27 patients aged 15 to 50 years and attributed this success to the application of an institutional protocol of "immediate reduction" (within 8 hours of diagnosis) and internal fixation with compression. This pivotal publication labeled these injuries "surgical emergencies" in young patients.

[a] Department of Orthopaedic Surgery, Lawrence J. Ellison Ambulatory Care Center, University of California, Davis, 4860 Y Street, Suite 3800, Sacramento, CA 95817, USA
[b] Department of Orthopaedic Surgery, University of Missouri, One Hospital Drive, MC213, Columbia, MO 65212, USA
[c] Division of Orthopaedic Surgery, Department of Surgery, McMaster University, Hamilton Health Sciences—General Site, 6 North Trauma, 237 Barton Street East, Hamilton, Ontario, Canada
* Corresponding author.
E-mail address: taniaferguson@ucdmc.ucdavis.edu

Orthop Clin N Am 41 (2010) 157–166
doi:10.1016/j.ocl.2010.01.001
0030-5898/10/$ – see front matter © 2010 Published by Elsevier Inc.

More recent evidence from cohort studies, however, does not conclusively support the association between time to reduction (<24 hours) and AVN. On one hand, Jain and colleagues[4] supported Swiontkowski's findings when they reported an increased rate of AVN (16%) in 38 patients (aged <60 years) treated more than 12 hours after injury and 0% AVN in patients treated within 12 hours of injury. On the other hand, Haidukewych and colleagues[5] retrospectively reviewed a series of 73 patients (aged 15–50 years) and found no significant difference in AVN in those treated within 24 hours of injury (23%) and those treated more than 24 hours after injury (20%). Three cases series reported that patients treated after inadvertent delays of 6 days to 2 years had rates of AVN similar to those series in which patients were treated emergently (0%–25%).[6–8]

To further support the lack of association between surgical timing and AVN, a meta-analysis was performed reviewing 18 retrospective cohort studies of femoral neck fractures in patients aged 15 to 50 years (547 fractures).[9] The overall rate of AVN for displaced fractures was 22.5%. Seven of these studies reported data on the association between surgical timing and AVN rates and demonstrated no difference between patients treated within 12 hours of injury (13.6%) and those treated after 12 hours of injury (15%). The only prospective data to date included 92 patients and demonstrated an overall AVN rate of 16%, with no difference in those patients treated before or after 48 hours at 2-year follow-up.[10]

Nonunion

Swiontkowski and colleagues[3] reported no nonunions in 27 patients and attributed this success to emergent surgical intervention, anatomic reduction, and compressive fixation. Jain and colleagues[4] reported no nonunions regardless of surgical delays of more than 12 hours. Haidukewych and colleagues[5] showed no difference in nonunion (overall rate 8%) seen in patients treated before or after 24 hours. Upadhyay and colleagues[10] found an overall nonunion rate of 17.4%, with no difference between those treated before or after 48 hours. The above-mentioned meta-analysis reported a 6% overall nonunion rate and found no significant difference between fractures treated within 12 hours (11.8%) or after 12 hours (5%) of injury.[9]

SHOULD THE INTRACAPSULAR PRESSURE/HEMATOMA BE DECOMPRESSED?

Although experimental data demonstrate an increase in the intracapsular hip pressure associated with femoral neck fractures,[11–14] there have not been any significant clinical benefits associated with capsulotomy. Maruenda and colleagues[14] prospectively measured preoperative intracapsular pressures in 34 patients with femoral neck fractures and observed the patients for an average of 7 years postoperatively. Five of the six patients in whom AVN developed had preoperative intracapsular pressures less than the diastolic blood pressure that led the investigators to conclude that the rate of AVN was not secondary to high intracapsular pressures. Upadhyay and colleagues[10] prospectively randomized patients to either closed reduction and percutaneous pinning or open capsulotomy, reduction, and pinning and found no difference in the rates of AVN and nonunion between treatment groups.

WHICH IMPLANT IS BEST FOR FEMORAL NECK FRACTURES IN YOUNG PATIENTS?

Femoral neck fracture fixation ideally allows interfragmentary compression, resists displacement, and ensures rotational stability during the healing process. Options for the fixation of femoral neck fractures include multiple compression screws (CSs), dynamic fixed-angle devices such as sliding hip screw (SHS) and side plate, static fixed-angle devices such as blade plate, dynamic condylar screw (DCS), and more recently, locked plates contoured to the proximal femur. The CS and the SHS constructs may allow fracture fragments to slide along the implants with axial loading during weight bearing and add the benefit of controlled dynamic compression during healing. Static fixed-angle devices aim to maintain the surgically obtained reduction rigidly during the healing period.

Although multiple clinical trials have directly compared implant choice with patient outcomes, these studies have all been performed in the osteoporotic patient population. Close evaluation of the small cohort studies of patients younger than 50 years of age demonstrate that most surgeons treat patients in this age group with various CS configurations; none of these studies specifically evaluate the association between nonunion and AVN with the fixation device. Moreover, complications of uncontrolled sliding with multiple screws and resultant shortening of the femoral neck are well reported in older patients but have not been critically evaluated in younger populations with good bone quality.

The biomechanical principles of fixation devices apply regardless of patient age. When using CSs, it is important to place them parallel to achieve compression[3] and close to the cortex to minimize the risk of nonunion and to prevent postoperative varus angulation and posteroinferior displacement of the femoral head.[15] Eighty-nine percent of fractures fixed with 2 screws placed within 3 mm of the inferior neck cortex and the posterior calcar region achieved union, but there was a 100% nonunion rate if both screws were more than 3 mm away from the cortices.[15]

The Pauwel classification is most commonly used for the evaluation of the young patient and is based on the biomechanical properties associated with the angle of the primary fracture line relative to the horizontal. In Pauwel type I fractures (<30°), compressive forces predominate, and screw position perpendicular to the fracture is often achievable. As the fracture becomes more vertical, shear forces predominate and it becomes more difficult to apply fixation perpendicular to the fracture line. A recent evaluation by Liporace and colleagues[16] retrospectively evaluated 62 young patients (19–64 years, mean age 42 years) with Pauwel type III fractures (>70°). Thirty-seven patients were treated with CS fixation and had a nonunion rate of 19%. The remaining 25 patients were treated with a fixed-angle implant (DCS, SHS, or cephalomedullary nail) and had an 8% rate of nonunion. Although sample size was small and there was no statistically significant difference because of insufficient power, this retrospective cohort study demonstrates the challenge of treating these high-shear fracture patterns in young patients and emphasizes the potential advantage of fixed-angle implants.

Poor reduction, typically varus malreduction, and posteroinferior displacement of the femoral head have been shown to increase the rate of nonunion irrespective of implant choice and patient age. Haidukewych and colleagues[5] reported an 80% nonunion rate in patients with a poor reduction versus 4% in those in whom a good to excellent reduction was achieved. Similarly, Liporace and colleagues[16] demonstrated a 14% nonunion rate in fractures with good to excellent reductions versus 2 of the 3 with poor reductions. Upadhyay and colleagues[10] prospectively associated nonunion with poor reduction, posterior neck comminution, and poor screw position. The presence of posterior neck comminution may compromise the surgeon's ability to obtain and maintain an anatomic reduction and has been associated with a lower resistance to displacement and fixation failure.[1,17,18]

SUMMARY OF THE EVIDENCE: PHYSIOLOGICALLY YOUNG PATIENTS

The goal of treatment in young patients is anatomic reduction and stable fixation of the femoral neck to minimize the risk of nonunion and osteonecrosis. Current best evidence suggests a lack of association between time to reduction (<24 hours) and AVN or nonunions. Similarly, although increased intracapsular pressure is associated with femoral neck fracture, no clinical benefit has been seen when capsular decompression is performed. The evidence, comprised of underpowered observational cohorts (level III–IV), is far from conclusive, and statistically sound inferences regarding surgical timing and capsular decompression cannot be made.

Regarding implant choice, the relative importance of dynamic compression during weight bearing at the cost of stability in unstable fracture patterns has not been evaluated. Although the theoretical benefit of fixed-angle implants should be considered in high-shear fractures (Pauwel III), an advantage over multiple screw fixation has not been clearly demonstrated in population-based studies. Although multiple screw fixation remains the current standard, trends favoring fixed-angle implants in the younger population demonstrate the need for ongoing comparative studies to ensure best practice. Quality of fracture reduction and presence of posterior comminution have been consistently associated with poor outcomes in young patients.

EXPERT OPINION

Femoral neck fracture reduction and fixation is indicated in patients with no evidence of osteopenia and who are poor candidates for hip replacement based on activity level. That said, indications for the fixation of femoral neck fractures have been affected by the improvements made in total hip replacement, which continues to grow as a treatment option for this injury with excellent results even in patients as young as 50 years old. Based on the evidence, the authors think strongly that if fixation is the goal, an anatomic reduction and rigid fixation are critical. All efforts should be put toward improving the likelihood of an anatomic reduction, and in our hands, an open reduction often improves the likelihood that this goal is achieved. Thus, an incision is preformed in the situation in which an anatomic reduction cannot be obtained closed, not necessarily as a method to decrease the risk of AVN. Notably, in the investigators' hands, an incision is often required to enhance reduction quality. The authors do not yet understand the importance of dynamic compression (afforded by CS or SHS fixation) on healing and think there may be some relevance to the consideration of fixed-angle implants in length-unstable fracture patterns, which fractures with comminution often are. However, the authors remain concerned that the locked implants, which create a bridge construct through the comminuted neck region, may lead to increased rates of nonunion because of the lack of compression and the rigidity created by these implants. The authors eagerly await further data on this topic. Finally, their interpretation of the available data indicates a lack of association between time to reduction and AVN or nonunions. Because these data are not definitive and low-level evidence, the current opinion remains that early reduction is the standard of care. The authors' practices include an assumption that quality of reduction is the most important factor on outcome, and if a surgical delay of 12 hours from injury enhances the likelihood of an anatomic reduction based on institutional factors, they would wait to perform the operation.

FEMORAL NECK FRACTURES IN OLD PATIENTS

Femoral neck fractures are significantly more common in the elderly than in physiologically young patients. Current projections suggest that 77 million Americans and 25% of Canadians will be older than 65 years by the year 2041.[19,20] It is predicted that Canadian and American health care systems will face the fiscal and social dilemma of 88,000 and 500,000 hip fractures a year, respectively.[19,20] Older patients are more likely to present with medical comorbidities; thus controversies regarding surgical timing are related to perioperative medical problems and mortality. Surgical controversies in this patient demographic include the benefit of fixation versus arthroplasty, implant options for internal fixation, and choices between partial and total hip arthroplasty.

IS THERE A ROLE FOR NONOPERATIVE MANAGEMENT IN THE ELDERLY WITH FEMORAL NECK FRACTURES?

Reported nonoperative protocols for hip fractures include a 1- to 3-week period of bed rest, followed by early bed-to-chair transfers and ambulation.[21,22] This treatment protocol has been associated with a 14% to 62% incidence of secondary displacement[11,23,24] versus 4.3% for similar fractures treated surgically.[12] Furthermore, the initial period of immobilization is associated with medical complications, including urinary tract infections, thromboembolic events, decubitus ulcers, and pneumonia.[21,22,25] Patients with cognitive dysfunction are at increased risk for complications associated with nonoperative treatment

(50% mortality and 63% complication).[13,26] Thus, although conservative management may be considered in high-risk surgical patients, it should be recognized that this option is associated with high rates of subsequent displacement, morbidity, and mortality.

Does Time to Surgery Matter?

Hip fractures in the elderly patient population are associated with an overall mortality rate averaging 30%.[27] Although several studies have demonstrated a direct correlation between surgical timing and patient mortality,[25,28–33] it is clear that patient comorbidities must be considered. Bottle and Aylin[32] recently reviewed patients older than 65 years (n = 129,522) and found that a delay in surgery of more than 24 hours was associated with increased inhospital death odds ratio of 1.39 (95% confidence interval [CI], 1.34–1.44). When comorbidities were controlled, the odds ratio fell to 1.27 (95% CI, 1.23–1.32). The investigators concluded that the presence of comorbidities does affect patient treatment, including time to surgery, but delay of surgery increases mortality and therefore should only be delayed secondary to optimization of comorbidities for surgery.

Radcliff and colleagues[33] prospectively analyzed patient outcomes in 5683 American veterans (aged >65 years) with femoral neck fractures and found that preinjury factors included older age, disseminated cancer, cognitive impairment, congestive heart failure, greater functional dependence, and higher ASA (III and IV). When these covariates were controlled, surgical delay more than 4 days was associated with increased 1-month mortality (odds ratio, 1.29; 95% CI, 1.02–1.61) as was the use of general anesthesia (odds ratio, 1.27; 95% CI, 1.15–1.53). They concluded that surgical delay of more than 4 days increased 1-month mortality.

Because surgical timing does seem to affect mortality, recent investigations have attempted to elucidate the optimal timing of surgical intervention in those patients presenting with medical conditions that may benefit from medical intervention before operation. Moran and colleagues[28] prospectively compared mortality rates at 1 month, 3 months, and 1 year among patients who were either fit for surgery or who required preoperative management of medical disease (n = 2660). Patients who were fit for surgery at the time of presentation but experienced surgical delay more than 4 days had increased 90-day (hazard ratio of 2.25; 95% CI, 1.2–4.3) and 1-year (hazard ratio of 2.4; 95% CI, 1.45–3.99) mortality rates. Patients with medical comorbidities requiring treatment had mortality rates 2.5 times higher than the fit cohort. Surgical delay did not influence the nonfit cohort's mortality rate. These data suggest that patients with treatable medical comorbidities have a significantly higher risk of overall mortality regardless of surgical timing and that priority should be given to optimizing medical management at the cost of surgical delay.

A meta-analysis of 16 prospective and retrospective observational studies demonstrated that surgical delay of more than 48 hours increased the 30-day and 1-year mortality rates by 41% and 32%, respectively.[30] The investigators concluded that for every 1000 patients undergoing delayed surgery versus early surgery, there would be 25 more deaths at 1 month and 49 at 1 year. Although all studies were observational, the sample sizes were high, and their findings were consistent with most large, population-based evaluations[28,30–32] that suggest a strong relationship among time to surgery, presence of medical comorbidities, and mortality (**Table 1**).

Which is Better: Internal Fixation or Arthroplasty?

Bone quality seems to be a significant factor in determining the success of internal fixation. Elderly patients with osteoporosis and poor bone quality have a higher risk of nonunion[34] (rates >30% in a large meta-analysis)[35] when treated with operative fixation of the femoral neck. Recent work by Zlowodzki and colleagues[36,37] demonstrated that union alone does not preclude a good functional outcome. Evaluation of 127 femoral neck fractures, 64% of which were nondisplaced at presentation, demonstrated a 66% incidence of shortening and a 39% incidence of varus collapse at the time of union. Femoral neck shortening of more than 5 mm correlated with decreased functional outcomes and, when combined with varus collapse, predicted the need for an assistive walking device. In a prospective randomized trial comparing internal fixation and arthroplasty, Ravikumar and Marsh[38] demonstrated a progressive decline in pain control and function during a 13-year period after successful internal fixation. In the first postoperative year, 88% of patients with internal fixation required no analgesia, compared with 33.3% at 13 years, and a total of 33% required revision surgery, which was compared with a 6.75% revision rate for total joint replacement.

Given the high rate of complications associated with internal fixation of femoral neck fractures, hip arthroplasty has become an increasingly important alternative in this patient demographic. A recent international surgeon survey revealed that most surgeons prefer internal fixation for younger patients (<60 years) and elderly patients with nondisplaced fractures (Garden type I).[27] However,

Table 1
Surgical timing in elderly hip fractures

Author	Study Design	Level of Evidence	Number	Summary
Zuckerman et al,[29] 1995	Prospective observation	B	367	Surgical delay >48 h doubled 1-y mortality (hazard ratio 1.76)
Moran et al,[28] 2005	Prospective observation	B	2660	Fit for surgery patients at presentation and surgical delay >4 d demonstrated increased 90-d (hazard ratio of 2.25; 95% CI, 1.2–4.3) and 1-y mortality rates (hazard ratio of 2.4; 95% CI, 1.45–3.99)
Bottle and Aylin,[32] 2006	Retrospective review	B	129,522	Delay in surgery >24 h was associated with increased inhospital death odds ratio 1.39 (95% CI, 1.34–1.44), and when comorbidities were controlled, the odds ratio fell to 1.27 (95% CI, 1.23–1.32)
Radcliff et al,[33] 2008	Prospective observation	B	5683	Surgical delay of >4 d after admission were associated with an increased risk of death within the first 30 d (odds ratio 1.29; 95% CI, 1.02–1.61)
Shiga et al,[30] 2008	[1]Meta-analysis	B	257,367	Surgical delay of >48 h increased the 30-d and 1-y mortality rates by 41% (odd ratio 1.41; 95% CI, 1.29–1.54) and 32% (odds ratio 1.32; 95% CI, 1.21–1.43)

most respondents preferred arthroplasty in Garden types III and IV (94% and 96%, respectively) in patients older than 80 years. Responses were significantly more variable when the 60- to 80-year-old patients with displaced femoral neck fractures were considered.

Many small clinical studies aimed at determining the risks and benefits of arthroplasty versus internal fixation in elderly patients with displaced femoral neck fractures have been performed in the last decade but have been underpowered.[39–43] The current best evidence comes from several excellent meta-analyses of randomized controlled trials published in the last 5 years.[42,44] These meta-analyses all demonstrate an increased risk of reoperation associated with internal fixation (weighted mean 35%) compared with arthroplasty (9%).[43] Two highly powered meta-analyses gave divergent results when evaluating the risks of complications and mortality associated with these 2 treatment methods (internal fixation vs arthroplasty). The meta-analysis by Bhandari and colleagues[42] (14 randomized trials, 1901 patients) found significantly higher rates in infection, blood loss, and an insignificant trend toward higher mortality at 4 months, whereas Rogmark and Johnell's[44] evaluation of 14 randomized trials comprising 2289 patients showed fewer complications with primary arthroplasty and no difference in mortality (**Table 2**).

Cost-analysis evaluations report that revision surgery associated with internal fixation is responsible for a greater fiscal expense compared with primary arthroplasty. Iorio and colleagues[46] compared outcomes and cost of 123 elderly patients treated with internal fixation, hemiarthroplasty, or total hip arthroplasty. Taking into consideration the reoperations, total hip arthroplasty ($20,670) was more cost-effective than internal fixation ($24,606). Keating and colleagues[47] evaluated functional outcomes and total cost of 207 elderly hip fractures in a prospective randomized trial. They reported that internal fixation was initially cheaper than arthroplasty but cumulative additional cost during a 2-year period after fixation resulted in a £3504 higher cost than bipolar or total joint replacement (95% CI, £1159–£5851). Heetveld and colleagues'[43] meta-analysis reported a similar increase in total costs associated with internal fixation.

WHAT IS THE BEST IMPLANT FOR INTERNAL FIXATION IN THE ELDERLY PATIENT POPULATION?

When internal fixation is determined to be a patient's best treatment option, a specific implant must be chosen. The biomechanical and technical principles remain the same as those reported previously for young patients. Parker and Blundell[48] conducted a meta-analysis of 25 randomized trials comparing different methods of fixation in 4925 elderly patients. They found no difference between fracture healing or complication rates of CS and SHS. Results from the meta-analysis by Bhandari and colleagues[42] demonstrated a significantly higher relative risk of revision surgery with multiple screw fixation when compared with a CS and side-plate construct, suggesting a benefit to using SHSs. A large multinational trial is currently underway to evaluate the efficacy of screws versus SHSs in patients with femoral neck fractures (Fixation using Alternative Implants for the Treatment of Hip Fractures [FAITH] trial). The trial aims to recruit

Table 2
Internal fixation versus arthroplasty

Author	Study Design	Level of Evidence	Number	Summary
Bhandari et al,[42] 2003	[2]Meta-analysis	A	301	Relative risk reduction for revision for arthroplasty 0.23; 95% confidence interval, 0.13–0.42; $P = .0003$
Blomfeldt et al,[39] 2005	[6]PRCT	A	102	4% complication rate for replacement vs 42% for fixation, $P<.001$. Four percent reoperation rates for replacement vs 47% for fixation
Bjorgul et al,[45] 2006	Prospective non-randomized	B	638	2% revision rate after hemiarthroplasty vs 24% for fixation, $P<.001$
Rogmark and Johnell,[44] 2006	[3]Meta-analysis	A	2289	Treatment related complication of ratio of 0.12 (95% CI, 0.09–0.15) for arthroplasty vs fixation

Abbreviation: PRCT, prospective, randomized controlled trial.

2500 patients with femoral neck fractures to determine the utility of SHSs in reducing revision surgeries and improving patient function.

WHAT TYPE OF ACUTE ARTHROPLASTY IS THE BEST FOR FEMORAL NECK FRACTURES?

When arthroplasty is the preferred procedure, implant decisions balance concerns over dislocation with total hip replacement[27] and acetabular wear with hemiarthroplasty. Ravikumar and Marsh[38] demonstrated that hemiarthroplasty was associated with greater pain (45% vs 6%), decreased mobility (53% vs 70%), lower Harris Hip Scores (55 vs 80), and higher revision rates than total hip arthroplasty (24% vs 6.75%). Keating and colleageus[47] evaluated patient-assessed outcomes between hemiarthroplasty and total hip replacement at 24 months, demonstrating a statistically significant improvement in hip rating questionnaire ($P<.04$) and a general level of health on the EQ-5D ($P<.008$) with total hip arthroplasty. Blomfeldt and colleagues[49] prospectively randomized 120 patients to primary total hip arthroplasty or hemiarthroplasty for the treatment of displaced femoral neck fractures. They reported a significant improvement in Harris Hip Scores at 4 and 12 months ($P = .011$ and $P<.001$) with total hip replacement and no significant differences in overall complications or mortality rates between treatment groups. The investigators concluded that total joint replacement was the preferred method of treatment for elderly, functionally independent patients who did not suffer from cognitive dysfunction.[38,43,44,47,49,50] Based on available evidence,

total hip arthroplasty is the preferred treatment for elderly, functionally independent patients, and hemiarthroplasty is reserved for demented patients. As an example, **Figs. 1** and **2** illustrate injury radiographs of 2 octogenarians. The patient illustrated in **Fig. 1** is an 84-year-old woman with stable coronary artery disease who is functionally independent and ambulates 1 mile a day. Based on her level of physical and mental function, a total hip arthroplasty was selected for her. On the other extreme, the images in **Fig. 2** represent an injury sustained by an 88-year-old woman who is a limited community ambulator with cane assist and suffers from multiple medical comorbidities. It was the investigator's opinion that this patient would best be served with a hemiarthroplasty given her limited ambulatory status (see **Figs. 1** and **2**; **Table 3**).

SUMMARY OF THE EVIDENCE: PHYSIOLOGICALLY OLDER PATIENTS

Femoral neck fractures in elderly patients represent a problem of epidemic proportion that will continue to grow substantially. They represent a major challenge technically and an enormous financial burden to patients and the health care system. Despite advances in contemporary management strategies, mortality rates in this patient cohort remain high (30%). There is a general consensus regarding operative intervention for all fractures of the femoral neck, because nonoperative management leads to high levels of disability, medical complications, and mortality. Surgical delays in fit patients without active

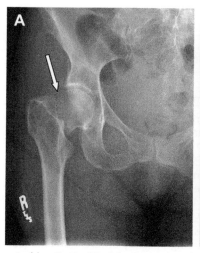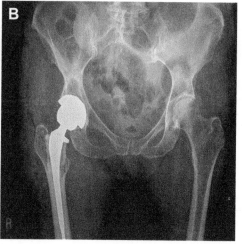

Fig. 1. 84-year-old patient with right femoral neck fracture. Functionally independent. (*A*) Preoperative anteroposterior (AP) right hip with femoral neck fracture (*white arrow*). (*B*) Postoperative AP pelvis with cemented total hip arthroplasty.

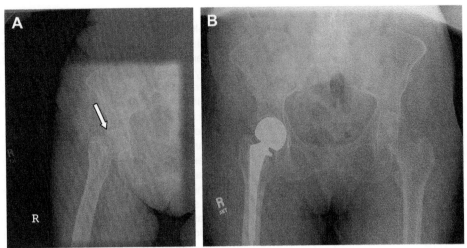

Fig. 2. 88-year-old limited community ambulatory patient with multiple medical comorbidities. (A) Preoperative anteroposterior (AP) right hip with femoral neck fracture (*white arrow*). (B) Postoperative AP pelvis with right cemented hemiarthroplasty.

medical issues result in an increase in mortality rates, although the ideal timing of surgery is patient-dependent and has not been clearly delineated. Patients with active medical issues should be optimized before surgery.

Internal fixation has a high rate of nonunion and fixation failure, and these rates are likely dependent on the underlying bone quality and fracture pattern. Although arthroplasty may decrease the rate of reoperation and improve functional results, this may come at the cost of increased infection rates and higher blood loss. Although most data do not show a difference in 1-year mortality rates regardless of treatment, the evidence comparing

internal fixation and arthroplasty consists of small randomized trials. Currently, treatment decisions are based on this body of evidence until larger multicenter randomized trials (Hip Fracture Evaluation with Alternatives of Total Hip Arthroplasty vs Hemiarthroplasty [HEALTH] and FAITH trials) are completed. Finally, although fixation constructs all seem to have similar complication rates, there is increasing evidence suggesting that total hip replacement improves patient functional outcomes compared with hemiarthroplasty for healthy, independent, elderly patients and should be considered as the treatment of choice for these patients.

Table 3
Hemiarthroplasty versus total hip arthroplasty in the elderly

Author	Study Design	Level of Evidence	Number	Summary
Ravikumar and Marsh,[38] 2000	PRCT	A	290	Patient reported significant pain at 13 y for hemiarthroplasty (45%) vs total hip (0%). Harris Hip Scores at 13 y for hemiarthroplasty (55) vs total hip (80)
Keating et al,[47] 2006	PRCT	B	207	A significant improvement in hip rating questionnaire ($P<.04$) and general level of health on the EQ-5D ($P<.008$) in favor of total hip was documented at 24 mo
Blomfeldt et al,[49] 2007	PRCT	A	120	Harris Hip Scores for [4]THA and hemiarthroplasty were significantly different at 4 mo (82.5 and 77.5, $P = .011$) and 12 mo (87.2 and 79.4, $P<.001$)

Abbreviation: PRCT, prospective, randomized controlled trial.

REFERENCES

1. Ly TV, Swiontkowski MF. Treatment of femoral neck fractures in young adults. Instr Course Lect 2009; 58:69–81.
2. Hirose J, Mizuta H, Ide J, et al. Evaluation of estimation of physiologic ability and surgical stress (E-PASS) to predict the postoperative risk for hip fracture in elder patients. Arch Orthop Trauma Surg 2008;128:1447–52.
3. Swiontkowski MF, Winquist RA, Hansen ST Jr. Fractures of the femoral neck in patients between the ages of twelve and forty-nine years. J Bone Joint Surg Am 1984;66(6):837–46.
4. Jain R, Koo M, Kreder HJ, et al. Comparison of early and delayed fixation of subcapital hip fractures in patients sixty years of age or less. J Bone Joint Surg Am 2002;84(9):1605–12.
5. Haidukewych GJ, Rothwell WS, Jacofsky DJ, et al. Operative treatment of femoral neck fractures in patients between the ages of fifteen and fifty years. J Bone Joint Surg Am 2004;86(8):1711–6.
6. Butt MF, Dhar SA, Gani NU, et al. Delayed fixation of displaced femoral neck fractures in younger adults. Injury 2008;39(2):238–43.
7. Huang CH. Treatment of neglected femoral neck fractures in young adults. Clin Orthop Relat Res 1986;206:117–26.
8. Roshan A, Ram S. Early return to function in young adults with neglected femoral neck fractures. Clin Orthop Relat Res 2006;447:152–7.
9. Damany DS, Parker MJ, Chojnowski A. Complications after intracapsular hip fractures in young adults. A meta-analysis of 18 published studies involving 564 fractures. Injury 2005;36(1):131–41.
10. Upadhyay A, Jain P, Mishra P, et al. Delayed internal fixation of fractures of the neck of the femur in young adults. A prospective, randomised study comparing closed and open reduction. J Bone Joint Surg Br 2004;86(7):1035–40.
11. Holmberg S, Kalén R, Thorngren KG. Treatment and outcome of femoral neck fractures. An analysis of 2418 patients admitted from their own homes. Clin Orthop Relat Res 1987;218:42–52.
12. Conn KS, Parker MJ. Undisplaced intracapsular hip fractures: results of internal fixation in 375 patients. Clin Orthop Relat Res 2004;421:249–54.
13. Ooi LH, Wong TH, Toh CL, et al. Hip fractures in nonagenarians: a study on operative and non-operative management. Injury 2005;36:142–7.
14. Maruenda JI, Barrios C, Gomar-Sancho F. Intracapsular hip pressure after femoral neck fracture. Clin Orthop Relat Res 1997;340:172–80.
15. Lindequist S. Cortical screw support in femoral neck fractures: a radiographic analysis of 87 fractures with a new mensuration technique. Acta Orthop Scand 1993;64(3):289–93.
16. Liporace F, Gaines R, Collinge C, et al. Results of internal fixation of Pauwels type-3 vertical femoral neck fractures. J Bone Joint Surg Am 2008;90(8): 1654–9.
17. Bosch U, Schreiber T, Krettek C. Reduction and fixation of displaced intracapsular fractures of the proximal femur. Clin Orthop Relat Res 2002;399:59–71.
18. Scheck M. Intracapsular fractures of the femoral neck. Comminution of the posterior neck cortex as a cause of unstable fixation. J Bone Joint Surg Am 1959;41:1187–200.
19. Cummings SR, Rubin SM, Black D. The future of hip fractures in the United States. Numbers, cost, and potential effects of post-menopausal estrogen. Clin Orthop Relat Res 1990;252:163–6.
20. Papadimitropoulos EA, Coyte PC, Josse RG, et al. Current and projected rates of hip fracture in Canada. CMAJ 1997;157(10):1357–63.
21. Tanaka J, Seki N, Tokimura F, et al. Conservative treatment of Garden stage I femoral neck fracture in elderly patients. Arch Orthop Trauma Surg 2002; 122:24–8.
22. Goldstein CB, Ferguson T, Bhandari M, et al. Implants for fixation of femoral neck fractures. Tech Orthop 2008;23(4):301–8.
23. Raaymakers EM, Marti RK. Non-operative treatment of impacted femoral neck fractures. A prospective study of 170 cases. J Bone Joint Surg Br 1991; 73(6):950–4.
24. Hansen FF. Conservative vs surgical treatment of impacted, subcapital fractures of the femoral neck. Acta Orthop Scand Suppl 1994;256:9.
25. Egol KA, Strauss EJ. Perioperative considerations in geriatric patients with hip fractures: what is the evidence? J Orthop Trauma 2009;23(6):386–94.
26. Sherk HH, Snape WJ, Loprete FL. Internal fixation versus nontreatment of hip fractures in senile patients. Clin Orthop Relat Res 1979;280:196–8.
27. Bhandari M, Devereaux PJ, Tornetta P 3rd, et al. Operative management of displaced femoral neck fractures in elderly patients. An international survey. J Bone Joint Surg Am 2005;87(9):2122–30.
28. Moran CG, Wenn RT, Sikand M, et al. Early mortality after hip fracture: is delay before surgery important? J Bone Joint Surg Am 2005;87(3):483–9.
29. Zuckerman JD, Skovron ML, Koval KJ, et al. Postoperative complications and mortality associated with operative delay in older patients who have a fracture of the hip. J Bone Joint Surg Am 1995;77(10):1551–6.
30. Shiga T, Wajima Z, Ohe Y. Is operative delay associated with increased mortality of hip fracture patients? Systematic review, meta-analysis, and meta-regression. Can J Anesth 2008;55(3):146–54.
31. Hommel A, Ulander K, Bjorkelund KB, et al. Influence of optimized treatment of people with hip fracture on time to operation, length of hospital stay,

reoperations and mortality within 1 year. Injury 2008; 39:1164–74.

32. Bottle A, Aylin P. Mortality associated with delay in operation after hip fracture: observational study. BMJ 2006;332(7547):947–51.

33. Radcliff TA, Henderson WG, Stoner TJ, et al. Patient risk factors, operative care, and outcomes among older community-dwelling male veterans with hip fracture. J Bone Joint Surg Am 2008;90(1):34–42.

34. Hedstrom M. Are patients with a nonunion after a femoral neck fracture more osteoporotic than others? BMD measurement before the choice of treatment: a pilot study of hip BMD and biochemical bone markers in patients with femoral neck fractures. Acta Orthop Scand 2004;75(1):50–2.

35. Lu-Yao GL, Keller RB, Littenberg B, et al. Outcomes after displaced fractures of the femoral neck. A meta-analysis of one hundred and six published reports. J Bone Joint Surg Am 1994;76(1):15–25.

36. Zlowodzki M, Jonsson A, Paulke R, et al. Shortening after femoral neck fracture fixation: is there a solution? Clin Orthop Relat Res 2007;461:213–8.

37. Zlowodzki M, Brink O, Switzer J, et al. The effect of shortening and varus collapse of the femoral neck on function after fixation of intracapsular fracture of the hip. J Bone Joint Surg Br 2008;90(11):1487–94.

38. Ravikumar KJ, Marsh G. Internal fixation versus hemiarthroplasty versus total hip arthroplasty for displaced subcapital fractures of femur—13 year results of a prospective randomised study. Injury 2000;31:793–7.

39. Blomfeldt R, Törnkvist H, Ponzer S, et al. Comparison of internal fixation with total hip replacement for displaced femoral neck fractures. J Bone Joint Surg Am 2005;87(8):1680–8.

40. Swiontokowski MF, Harrington RM, Keller TS, et al. Torsion and bending anaylsis of internal fixation techniques for femoral neck fractures: the role of implant design and bone density. J Orthop Res 1987;5(3):433–44.

41. Rogmark C, Carlsson A, Johnell O, et al. A prospective randomised trial of internal fixation versus arthroplasty for displaced fractures of the neck of the femur. Functional outcome for 450 patients at two years. J Bone Joint Surg Br 2002;84(2):183–8.

42. Bhandari M, Devereaux PJ, Swiontkowski MF, et al. Internal fixation compared with arthroplasty for displaced fractures of the femoral neck. A meta-analysis. J Bone Joint Surg Am 2003;85(9):1673–81.

43. Heetveld MJ, Rogmark C, Frihagen F, et al. Internal fixation versus arthroplasty for displaced femoral neck fractures: what is the evidence? J Orthop Trauma 2009;23(6):395–402.

44. Rogmark C, Johnell O. Primary arthroplasty is better than internal fixation of displaced femoral neck fractures: a meta-analysis of 14 randomized studies with 2,289 patients. Acta Orthop Scand 2006;77(3):359–67.

45. Bjorgul K, Reikeras O. Hemiarthroplasty in worst cases is better than internal fixation in best cases of displaced femoral neck fractures: a prospective study of 683 patients treated with hemiarthroplasty or internal fixation. Acta Orthopaedica Scandinavica 2006;77(3):368–74.

46. Iorio R, Healy WL, Lemos DW, et al. Displaced femoral neck fractures in the elderly outcomes and cost effectiveness. Clin Orthop Relat Res 2001; 383:229–42.

47. Keating JF, Grant A, Masson M, et al. Randomized comparison of reduction and fixation, bipolar hemiarthroplasty, and total hip arthroplasty. Treatment of displaced intracapsular hip fractures in healthy older patients. J Bone Joint Surg Am 2006;88(2):249–60.

48. Parker MJ, Blundell C. Choice of implant for internal fixation of femoral neck fractures: meta-analysis of 25 randomised trials including 4,925 patients. Acta Orthop Scand 1998;69(2):138–43.

49. Blomfeldt R, Törnkvist H, Eriksson K, et al. A randomised controlled trial comparing bipolar hemiarthroplasty with total hip replacement for displaced intracapsular fractures of the femoral neck in elderly patients. J Bone Joint Surg Br 2007;89(2):160–5.

50. Schmidt AH, Leighton R, Parvizi J, et al. Optimal arthroplasty for femoral neck fractures: is total hip arthroplasty the answer? J Orthop Trauma 2009; 23(6):428–33.

Fusion Versus Disk Replacement for Degenerative Conditions of the Lumbar and Cervical Spine: Quid Est Testimonium?

Thomas J. Kishen, MBBS, DNB,
Ashish D. Diwan, MS, DNB, PhD*

KEYWORDS

- Cervical • Lumbar • Spinal fusion
- Intervertebral disk replacement

Quid est testimonium (in Latin, "what is the evidence")? With 70% of the population likely to have at least one episode of neck and back pain in their lives[1–4] it is not surprising that back pain is the second most common reason for visiting a family physician.[5] The natural history of low back pain points toward a high rate of recurrence and ongoing disability.[6,7] In addition to the suffering and disability, chronic spinal pain is associated with enormous direct and indirect costs.[8–11] Axial spinal pain can originate from degenerated intervertebral disks; facet joint arthritis; and secondarily from the muscles, ligaments, and neural tissue. Pain perception involves a complex interaction at multiple levels of the neural pathway with central modulation[12] and psychosocial factors influence the development and perpetuation of chronic pain.[13] Nonoperative modalities including physiotherapy, pain pharmacotherapy, and spinal injections are the first-line treatment options for chronic axial spinal pain. Spinal fusion and total disk replacement (TDR) can be considered for recalcitrant symptoms.

Lumbar TDR is indicated in the management of discogenic back pain without facet arthritis; however, 95% of potential surgical patients are likely to have a contraindication for lumbar TDR.[14,15] Lumbar fusion, however, has wider indications. In the cervical spine, anterior cervical diskectomy and fusion (ACDF) and TDR are advocated for radiculopathy and myelopathy with or without axial neck pain and nearly 50% of surgical patients with degenerative conditions qualify for a cervical TDR.[16] This article compares the outcomes of spinal fusion and disk replacement for degenerative conditions of the lumbar and cervical spine. Also discussed is the philosophy of the surgical management of degenerative conditions of the lumbar and cervical spine.

LUMBAR FUSION

Spinal fusion, first reported 100 years ago[17,18] for posttuberculosis spinal deformity, is now being used to manage trauma, deformity, instability, and degenerative conditions. Fusion for degenerative

Research and education funding has been received from Stryker and Synthes.
Spine Service, Department of Orthopedic Surgery, St George Hospital and Clinical School, University of New South Wales, 53 Montgomery Street, Kogarah, New South Wales 2217, Australia
* Corresponding author.
E-mail address: a.diwan@spine-service.org

Orthop Clin N Am 41 (2010) 167–181
doi:10.1016/j.ocl.2009.12.002

conditions is based on the premise that obliteration of movement and off-loading the diseased motion segment relieves pain. Spinal fusion, with or without supplementary instrumentation, can be performed through a posterior (posterolateral fusion, posterior lumbar interbody fusion, and transforaminal lumbar interbody fusion), anterior (anterior lumbar interbody fusion [ALIF]), or combined approach (anteroposterior fusion). In the 5-year period from 1996 to 2001, the number of lumbar fusions performed in the United States increased by 113% with more procedures being performed for degenerative conditions[19] and wide regional variations in the number and outcomes of lumbar fusion.[20]

Despite the increasing number of lumbar fusions being performed, there are numerous unresolved issues including the efficacy of the procedure, potential for accelerated adjacent level degeneration (ALD), pseudoarthrosis, and bone graft donor site morbidity. Stiff fusion constructs in the lumbar spine lead to abnormal stresses on the adjacent levels[21,22] potentially leading to accelerated ALD. Although the significance of radiologic ALD is unknown, the rate of symptomatic ALD requiring either decompression or fusion is predicted to be 17% at 5 years and 36% at 10 years following spinal fusion.[23] Nevertheless, the debate continues whether the ALD is in reality a natural progression of the degenerative process.

Wide variations in the rate of pseudoarthrosis (nonunion) have been reported (2.3%–83.3%) following lumbar fusion,[24] and can have a negative impact on the clinical outcome. Donor site morbidity at the bone graft harvest site[25] is another cause for concern. Alternatives to autograft, such as allograft[26,27] and bone morphogenetic protein (BMP),[28] have shown equivalent outcomes; however, the use of BMP increases the cost of the procedure substantially.[29] The efficacy of lumbar fusion for degenerative conditions is the major cause for concern, and in this context two issues need consideration.

What are the Outcomes of Lumbar Fusion for Degenerative Disease?

A review of literature[30] analyzed the influence of subdiagnosis on the outcome of lumbar fusion and found significantly better clinical outcomes for spondylolisthesis compared with degenerative disk disease. Buttermann and colleagues[31] reported satisfaction rates of 100%, 76%, and 69% in patients who underwent fusion for spondylolisthesis, disk degeneration, and postdiskectomy, respectively. Similarly, Glassman and colleagues[32] found that a higher percentage of

patients with spondylolisthesis attained minimum clinically important improvement for oswestry disability index (ODI) (71% vs 57%), back pain (60% vs 57%), and leg pain (63% vs 51%) compared with disk pathology following a posterolateral fusion. Slosar and colleagues[33] also reported higher satisfaction following circumferential spinal fusion in patients with listhesis and stenosis (80%) when compared with painful disk degeneration (56%) and internal disk disruption (50%). **Table 1** lists some of the studies relating to the outcomes following spinal fusion.

Several studies have reported better clinical outcomes following a circumferential fusion for patients with degenerative disk disease,[34–37] whereas others did not find any difference between various methods of fusion.[38] A meta-analysis of randomized controlled trials (RCT)[39] concluded that although circumferential fusion enhanced the fusion rate and reduced the reoperation rate, there was no significant difference in the global assessment of clinical outcomes compared with instrumented posterolateral fusion.

Are the Outcomes of Spinal Fusion Superior to Nonoperative Treatment?

Three RCTs found no significant difference when lumbar fusion was compared with a structured rehabilitation program using cognitive principles.[40–42] Fritzell and colleagues,[43] however, found lumbar fusion to be more efficacious than unstructured nonoperative therapy. Two reviews of RCTs comparing fusion with nonoperative treatment concluded that limitations in the RCTs prevented a definitive conclusion of comparative efficacy,[44,45] whereas another systematic review[46] concluded that fusion is no more effective than intensive rehabilitation but associated with small to moderate benefits compared with standard nonsurgical therapy. A meta-analysis of randomized trials[47] concluded that cumulative evidence did not support surgical fusion for the treatment for chronic low back pain. The details of studies comparing fusion with nonoperative treatment are given in **Table 2**.

The clinical outcomes following fusion for spondylolisthesis are favorable, whereas for lumbar disk degeneration, it is unclear whether fusion is more efficacious than a structured nonoperative program.

Lumbar TDR

Fernstrom's early attempts to retain segmental motion (1950s) using metallic balls led to subsidence because of the small area of contact and disparity in the modulus of elasticity between the

Table 1
List of review articles analyzing the outcomes following lumbar fusion

Authors	Study	Conclusion
Christensen, 2004[34] Review	9 studies (2 retrospective, 1 prospective, 5 RCT's, and 1 animal study)	Spondylolisthesis served better with noninstrumented posterolateral fusion; degenerative conditions better with anteroposterior fusion
Gibson and Waddell, 2005[80] Cochrane review	31 RCT's	Limited evidence to support surgery
Resnick et al, 2005[44] Review	2 RCT's and numerous case series and control studies	Insufficient evidence to support a treatment guideline for intractable low back pain without stenosis or spondylolisthesis
Mirza and Deyo, 2007[45] Systematic review	4 RCT's	Surgery may be more efficacious than unstructured nonsurgical care but may not be more than structured cognitive behavioral therapy; limitations of the RCT's prevent firm conclusions
Ibrahim et al, 2008[47] Meta-analysis	3 RCT's for primary analysis and 1 for sensitivity analysis	Evidence at present does not support routine surgical fusion for treatment of chronic low back pain
Carreon et al, 2008[81] Systematic review	25 studies	Spondylolisthesis did better than DDD following fusion; no difference in outcomes between different fusion procedures
Chou et al, 2009[46] Systematic review (American Pain Society Clinical Practice guidelines)	84 trials and 24 reviews	Fusion is no more effective than intensive rehabilitation but has small to moderate benefits compared with standard nonsurgical therapy; clinical benefits of instrumented versus noninstrumented fusion is unclear
Han et al, 2009[39] Meta-analysis	4 RCT's	No significant difference in clinical outcome between instrumented posterolateral fusion and circumferential fusion

Abbreviations: DDD, degenerative disk disease; RCTs, randomized controlled trials.

Table 2
Randomized controlled trials comparing lumbar fusion with nonoperative treatment

Authors and Type of Study	Sample Size and Follow-up	Outcomes	Comments
Fritzell et al, 2001[43] RCT	73 noninstrumented posterolateral fusion; 74 instrumented posterolateral fusion; 75 anteroposterior fusion (circumferential fusion); 72 nonoperative treatment Age: 25–65 y F/U : 2 y	Greater improvement in pain, disability, return to work, and satisfaction in surgical group; 63% of surgical patients improved compared with 29% nonoperative; 75% of surgery patients would go through procedure again compared with 53% of nonoperative	Nonoperative group had unstructured (usual care) therapy Listhesis, postdiskectomy, fractures, and infection excluded Various surgical procedures compared with nonoperative Data excluded crossover patients
Brox et al, 2003[42] RCT	37 instrumented posterolateral fusion versus 27 cognitive/exercises Age: 25–60 y F/U: 1 y	No difference in ODI, back pain, and general function between groups; leg pain improved in surgical group; 71% surgical and 63% nonoperative patients rated their outcomes as successful (not significant)	Nonoperative group had exercises and cognitive therapy Excluded: patients with stenosis, radiculopathy, and previous surgery Small sample
Fairbank et al, 2005[40] RCT	176 fusion versus 173 nonoperative treatment Age: 18–55 y F/U: 2 y	ODI: minor difference in favor of surgery SF-36: no difference Shuttle walk test: no difference between groups	Nonoperative group had exercises and cognitive therapy High drop-out and crossover rate Multiple diagnosis (listhesis, postlaminectomy, CLBP) Multiple surgical procedures including Graf stabilization
Brox et al, 2006[41] RCT	28 instrumented posterolateral fusion versus 29 nonoperative treatment for postdiskectomy back pain Age: 25–60 y F/U: 1 y	No significant difference in ODI scores Overall success rate: 50% (surgical) versus 48%	Nonoperative group had exercises and cognitive therapy Small numbers 97% follow-up Five patients did not attend treatment and two crossed over

Abbreviations: CLBP, chronic low back pain; ODI, oswestry disability index; RCTs, randomized controlled trials.

spherical prosthesis and flat bony end plates. Structural failure of the elastomeric-viscoelastic polyolefin rubber and silicon core attached to two titanium plates in the Acroflex prosthesis (Depuy, Acromed Corporation, Cleveland, OH, USA) was noticed during clinical trials. Among the numerous patented artificial intervertebral disk designs very few have undergone clinical trials.[48] The clinical outcomes following the implantation of two Food and Drug Administration (FDA) approved disk prosthesis are discussed next and are also listed in **Table 3**.

TDR, by restoring disk height, segmental lordosis, and segmental motion, can potentially reduce the risk of accelerated ALD. Biomechanical analysis has shown that the disk prosthesis preserved physiologic loading[21,22] at adjacent nonoperated levels compared with spinal fusion. A retrospective radiographic study of 42 patients followed for 8 years following lumbar TDR[49] showed that implanted prosthesis exhibiting greater than 5 degrees of motion revealed 0% and those with less than 5 degrees of motion showed a 34% incidence of ALD. TDR obviates the need for bone graft thereby avoiding donor site morbidity and the need for the expensive BMP to augment the fusion.

Charité Artificial Disk Prosthesis

Ninety percent of 100 patients implanted with the Charité III prosthesis (Depuy Spine, Raynham, MA, USA) reported good to excellent results (Modified Stauffer Coventry Scale) at 10 years with 80% returning to their previous employment.[50] Although no prosthesis failure was reported, five patients underwent a secondary fusion. David[51] reported the 10-year outcomes (mean follow-up, 13.2 years) following one-level disk arthroplasty with the Charité prosthesis in 106 patients. A total of 82% of the patients reported excellent or good clinical outcomes and 90% of implanted prostheses were mobile at the last follow-up. Eight patients (7.5%) underwent a posterior fusion at index level and three (2.8%) underwent adjacent-level surgery.

In the FDA investigational device exemption (FDA-IDE) study,[52] patients with single-level disk degeneration between L4 and S1 were randomized to undergo either a Charité prosthesis implantation (N = 205) or a stand-alone anterior fusion with cages and autograft (N = 99). Clinical success at 2 years, defined as absence device failure, major complications, or neurologic deterioration and greater than 25% improvement in ODI score, was achieved in 57% of TDR patients and 46% of the fusion group (P<.05). The study concluded that the 2-year clinical outcome was equivalent to anterior fusion and subsequently the Charité III device was approved by the FDA for implantation in patients with one-level disk degeneration from L4 to S1 who had failed at least 6 months of conservative treatment. Five-year follow-up of 90 Charité and 43 BAK fusion patients from the IDE study[53] (44% of initial cohort) showed an overall success rate of 57% and 51%, respectively (P = .0359). The improvement in the visual analogue scale (VAS) and ODI was similar in both groups at 2 and 5 years. The results at 5 years were similar to the 2-year results demonstrating noninferiority of the Charité group versus anterior fusion.

ProDisc-L Artificial Disk Prosthesis

Seven- to 11-year outcomes (mean, 8.7 years) following the ProDisc I implantation, in 55 out of 64 patients available for follow-up, showed 75% good to excellent results (relative improvement score >60%) and 64% were entirely satisfied with the results, whereas 5% were not satisfied.[54] No device failure or migration was noted. As part of the randomized FDA-IDE study, patients with single-level disk degeneration between L3 and S1 who underwent TDR with the ProDisc-L (Synthes Spine, West Chester, Pennsylvania) prosthesis (N = 161) were compared with those who underwent a circumferential spinal fusion (N = 75) and followed-up for 2 years.[55] Clinical success as defined by the FDA includes success for each individual case in the domains of ODI, SF-36, device-related, radiologic, and neurologic parameters, and was achieved in 41% of the fusion patients and 53% of the TDR patients. The study concluded that implantation of the ProDisc prosthesis was safe and superior to circumferential fusion using multiple clinical criteria. Subsequently, ProDisc-L was approved by the FDA in August 2006 for use in single-level disk degeneration between L3 and S1 following failure of 6 months of nonoperative management. A 3-year comparative analysis of the clinical outcomes (ODI, VAS, mean subjective improvement rate, and clinical success rate) following implantation of the ProDisc prosthesis and Charité prosthesis revealed similar results.[56]

Financial Implications: Lumbar Fusion Versus TDR

With burgeoning health care expenditure, cost-benefit analysis of new technology needs careful consideration. Costs vary between hospitals, regions, states, and countries. Guyer and coworkers[57] found that the hospital costs of ALIF plus autograft, ALIF plus BMP, and posterior lumbar interbody fusion were 12%, 36.5%, and 36.5% higher, respectively, compared with one-level TDR (Charité prosthesis) and concluded that the cost of a one-level TDR is less than or at worst equal to a one-level fusion. Another analysis of total hospital costs[58] (excluding BMP) for transforaminal lumbar interbody fusion ($29,260), ALIF ($26,767), and TDR $27,972 was roughly similar and lower than anteroposterior fusion ($39,233). With inclusion of the cost of BMP, however, the cost of TDR was significantly lower than the three fusion procedures (transforaminal lumbar interbody fusion, $34,660; ALIF, $32,167;

Table 3
List of studies analyzing the outcomes following lumbar total disk replacement

Author	Study	Outcome	Comments
Blumenthal et al, 2005[52] RCT	205 Charite TDR versus 99 ALIF Mean age: 39 y F/U: 2 y	No significant difference in VAS /ODI 73% (TDR) and 53% satisfaction 70% (TDR) and 50% would have procedure again (P<.05) 57% (TDR) and 46% clinical success (FDA criteria)	Industry sponsored Stand-alone ALIF Noninferiority study 11 TDR (5.4%) and 9 (9.1%) fusion patients underwent additional surgery at index level
Guyer et al, 2009[53] RCT	90 Charite TDR versus 43 ALIF Mean age: 39 y F/U: 5 y	No significant difference in VAS /ODI /SF-36 (PCS) 58% (TDR) and 51% clinical success (FDA criteria) 78% (TDR) and 72% of patients satisfied	Industry sponsored 43% lost to follow-up
David, 2007[51] Retrospective	108 one-level Charite TDR patients Mean age: 36 y F/U: 10 y	82% good-excellent outcome 89% return to work with 77% return to previous hard labor Mean flex-ext ROM = 10.1 degrees; 7.5% revision fusion; 8 patients (7.5%) underwent a posterior fusion at index level and 3 patients (2.8%) underwent adjacent level surgery (two disk herniation and one spinal canal stenosis)	106 patients available for follow-up

Study	Details	Results	Comments
Lemaire et al, 2005[50] Retrospective	107 Charite prosthesis (1–3 levels) Mean age: 39 y F/U: 10 y	90% good-excellent outcome, 91% of those eligible returned to work, mean flex-ext ROM = 10.3 degrees Minor posttraumatic subsidence (2), periprosthetic ossification (3), adjacent level degeneration (2) and requiring secondary fusion (5)	100 patients available for follow-up
Tropiano et al, 2005[54] Retrospective	64 ProDisc patients (1–3 level) Mean age: 46 y F/U: 8.7 y	75% good-excellent results; significant improvements in back and leg pain and disability	55 available for follow-up
Zigler et al, 2007[55] RCT	161 ProDisc TDR versus 75 APF (1–2 level) Mean age: 40 y F/U: 2 y	53% (TDR) and 40% success (FDA criteria) 81%(TDR) and 69% would have same procedure again No significant difference in ODI, pain, SF-36 scores	Industry sponsored 6 failures in TDR group: prosthesis migration (1), core migration (3), improper insertion of core (1), persistent pain requiring fusion (1)
Berg et al, 2009[82] RCT	80 TDR versus 72 fusion Age: 20–55 y F/U: 2 y	No significant difference in ODI, 84% (TDR) and 86%(fusion) improved, Minor difference in back and leg pain in favor of TDR	Three different prosthesis used and two fusion procedures (PLF, PLIF) Small numbers in each group

Abbreviations: ALIF, anterior lumbar interbody fusion; APF, anterior-posterior fusion; FDA, Food and Drug Administration; ODI, oswestry disability index; PCS, physical component scores; PLF, posterolateral fusion; PLIF, posterior lumbar interbody fusion; RCT, randomized controlled trial; TDR, total disk replacement; VAS, visual analogue scale.

Table 4
List of studies analyzing the outcomes following cervical total disk replacement

Authors and Study	Materials and Methods	Outcome	Comments
Anderson et al, 2004[83] Prospective BRYAN disk prosthesis	97 one-level and 39 two-level TDR F/U: 1 and 2 y	75 one-levels completed 2 y f/u 45 excellent, 7 good, 13 fair, and 8 poor 30 two-levels completed 1 year F/U: 21excellent, 3 good, 5 fair, and 1 poor Significant improvement in SF-36 scores for one- and two-levels	Early results from European trial
Sasso et al, 2007[72] RCT BRYAN disk prosthesis	56 TDR versus 59 ACDF Mean age: 42–46 y F/U: 2 y	TDR showed significant improvement in NDI, neck pain, and physical component score of SF-36 compared with ACDF Arm pain relief and Sf-36 (MCS) were similar	Subset of FDA trial 61% follow-up at 2 y 4 ACDF plus 3 TDR were reoperated ACDF: plate plus fibular allograft
Heidecke et al, 2008[84] Prospective BRYAN disk prosthesis	59 prosthesis in 54 patients (5 two-level) Mean age: 46 y Mean F/U: 2 y	43 excellent and 11 good outcome (Odoms) 12% had motion <3 degrees 29% had heterotrophic ossification	Mild postoperative kyphosis in first week after surgery
Heller et al, 2009[74] RCT BRYAN disk prosthesis	242 TDR versus 221 ACDF One-level Mean age: 44 y F/U: 2 y	NDI, neck pain score, and overall success were significantly better following TDR Arm pain score, SF-36, neurologic success, and return to work status were not statistically different Return to work was 2-week earlier in TDR group	ACDF: plate plus allograft 230 TDR and 194 ACDF available for 2 y F/U 94% successful fusion No spontaneous fusion in TDR group 117 patients refused participation after randomization

Study	Details	Results	Comments
Mummaneni et al, 2007[85] RCT (FDA-IDE) Prestige ST disk prosthesis	276 TDR versus 265 ACDF (single level) Mean age: 43 y F/U: 2 y	No significant difference in NDI, SF-36, neck and arm pain between groups Overall success and neurologic success were significantly higher in TDR group and a lower rate of adjacent level surgery	ACDF: ring allograft plus plate; 25% fusion, lost to F/U Revision surgery: 0 (TDR) and 5 (fusion) Adjacent level surgery: 3 (TDR group) and 11 procedures in 9 patients (fusion group) Hardware removal: 5 (TDR) and 9 (fusion)
Nabhan et al, 2007[76] RCT ProDisc-C disk prosthesis	25 TDR versus 24 ACDF (one-level) Mean age: 44 y F/U: 1 y	No significant difference in neck and arm pain between the two groups	Small numbers with short follow-u
Murrey et al, 2009[78] RCT, FDA ProDisc-C disk prosthesis	102 TDR versus 106 ACDF (one-level) Mean age: 43 y F/U: 2 y	No difference between groups in neurologic success, NDI scores, VAS scores, satisfaction, adverse events, SF36, and overall success	10% in each group had prior surgery 90% fusion following ACDF Higher rate of revisions following ACDF
Beaurain et al, 2009[86] Prospective Mobi-C disk prosthesis	85 prosthesis in 76 patients 67 one-level and 9 two-level Mean age: 43 y F/U: up to 2 y	Significant improvement in NDI and arm and neck pain VAS Improved return to work after surgery with reduced narcotic use 72% success rate and 91% would have the surgery again	12% had previous surgery 6/76 hybrid construct 11% had <3 degrees motion 9.1% adjacent level degeneration
Park et al, 2008[87] Retrospective Mobi-C disk prosthesis	21 TDR versus 32 ACDF (one-level) Mean age: 46 y F/U: 1 year	No difference in NDI, VAS, and satisfaction rate	Small numbers with short follow-up
Pimenta et al, 2007[88] Prospective PCM disk prosthesis	71 single level versus 69 multilevel TDR (229 levels in 140 patients) Mean age: 46 y F/U: 2 mo (26 mo)	Significantly better NDI and VAS scores in the multilevel group Success rate (Odom's) was 90.5% versus 93.9%	Reoperation rates and adverse events were similar between groups

Abbreviations: ACDF, anterior cervical diskectomy and fusion; FDA, Food and Drug Administration; IDE, investigational device exemption; NDI, neck disability index; RCT, randomized controlled trial; TDR, total disk replacement.

anteroposterior fusion, $44,633). Levin and coworkers[59] also studied the hospital costs and found similar implant cost for one-level TDR and circumferential fusion but higher operating room and surgeon charges for fusion resulted in a 23% higher cost for fusion surgery. In the two-level surgery group, the implant costs were lower in the fusion group ($18,460 vs $23,000) but there was no significant difference in the total cost. Similarly, an Australian federal government report did not find a significant difference in costs (hospitalization plus prosthesis plus medical fees) between fusion ($26,854 Australian dollars) and lumbar TDR ($24,139 Australian dollars).[60]

Summary: Lumbar Fusion Versus TDR

The short-term outcomes of lumbar TDR are equivalent to that following lumbar fusion. The cost of TDR in United States hospitals seems to be less than or equal to fusion. Lack of adequate long-term follow-up data prevents an analysis of the potential benefit of TDR in preventing or reducing the incidence of ALD.

CERVICAL SPINE

ACDF was described by Bailey and Badgley in 1939 and later modified by Cloward (1953) and Smith and Robinson (1955) to treat cervical radiculopathy or myelopathy with and without axial neck pain. Unlike the outcomes of fusion for lumbar degenerative disk disease, the outcomes following ACDF are generally favorable and range from 90% to 95% and are equivalent to hip arthroplasty.[61] Nevertheless, there are a few shortcomings including ALD, pseudoarthrosis, and donor site morbidity.

In vitro studies have shown increased segmental motion,[62,63] intradiscal pressure,[63,64] and facet forces[64] at levels adjacent to a cervical fusion construct. Goffin and coworkers[65] reported a 92% incidence of ALD 5 years after an ACDF with a 6% incidence of adjacent-level surgery following a failure to respond to nonoperative treatment. Hilibrand and coworkers[66] predicted a 25.6% incidence of symptomatic ALD within 10 years (2.9% per year) after an ACDF. A higher rate of ALD following one-level fusion compared with multilevel fusion, however, led the authors to believe that the changes were a natural progression of spondylosis rather than a consequence of surgery. Further, the 3.9% per year incidence of ALD, following noninstrumented posterior foraminolaminotomy,[67] is roughly equal to the incidence following ACDF. A prospective study[68] revealed significantly higher rates of radiologic ALD following an ACDF, however, compared with

TDR followed-up for 24 months. Additionally, a serial MRI study[69] showed increased disk degeneration adjacent to an ACDF compared with a posterior laminoplasty. The debate continues, however, on this subject.

In vitro studies showed that one- and two-level TDR, in addition to restoring motion at the index level, do not increase the motion at the adjacent levels,[70] thereby potentially reducing the incidence of ALD. TDR also precludes the need for autologous bone graft, avoiding bone graft donor site morbidity, which is a shortcoming of ACDF.

ACDF Versus Cervical TDR

Two-year follow-up of a randomized controlled trial[71] of 99 patients with one-level disk disease who underwent either ACDF or cervical TDR (Bryan artificial disk prosthesis, Medtronic Sofamor Danek, Memphis, TN, USA) from three participating centers of an FDA-IDE trial were reported. Significantly better outcomes in the domains of neck disability index, arm and neck pain, and the SF-36 physical component score were found in the TDR group. Revision surgery was performed in four patients from the fusion group for nonunion (N = 2) and ALD (N = 2) and two patients from the TDR group for ALD. The same authors[72] reported on the outcomes following an RCT with 2-year follow-up of 115 patients showing statistically better outcomes relating to neck disability index (NDI), neck pain, and SF-36 physical component score in the TDR group. Another participating center of the FDA-IDE trial[73] showed similar clinical outcomes in 33 patients with single-level disk disease randomized to have either ACDF (N = 16) or TDR (N = 17).

Heller and coworkers[74] reported the results of a multicenter RCT comparing TDR (Bryan disk prosthesis) (242 patients) with ACDF (221 patients) followed for 2 years. The patients who underwent TDR showed significantly better outcomes in the domains of NDI and neck pain but there was no difference between the two groups with regards to arm pain, SF-36 scores, neurologic success, and number of secondary surgical procedures. Overall success, as defined as greater than 15-point improvement in NDI scores, maintenance or improvement in neurologic status, absence of implant- or implant-surgical procedure–related serious adverse events, and absence of subsequent surgery or intervention, was statistically higher in the TDR group. An RCT comparing the outcomes of TDR (Bryan disk prosthesis) with ACDF in 65 patients with two-level disk disease[75] revealed significantly better outcomes in the TDR group with respect to NDI and arm and neck pain. In the TDR group, 29 patients reported good to excellent outcomes and one reported a fair outcome compared with 27 patients with good to excellent outcomes, fair outcomes in four patients, and poor outcomes in one patient.

Six-month and 1-year follow-up of an RCT comparing outcomes following single-level TDR (ProDisc-C, Synthes Spine, West Chester, PA, USA) with ACDF found similar improvements in arm and neck pain in both groups.[76,77] Murrey and coworkers[78] reported the outcome of an RCT comparing the outcomes of a single-level TDR (ProDisc-C) and ACDF. At the 2-year mark, there was no statistical difference between the two groups with relation to NDI, neurologic success, VAS score for neck and arm pain, SF-36, and patient satisfaction. A statistically higher proportion of the TDR patients reported overall success according to the FDA criteria and the minimally clinically important difference criteria. A few studies comparing the outcomes of TDR with ACDF are listed in **Table 4**.

Numerous RCTs have compared the outcomes of ACDF and cervical TDR. At this stage, some short-term results are favorable, whereas others show equivalence to cervical fusion. In the absence of long-term studies, the data on prosthesis survival and the effect of wear debris are unavailable.

Financial Implications: Cervical Fusion Versus TDR

Bhadra and colleagues,[79] from the United Kingdom, studied the clinical outcome and in-hospital costs of three ACDF methods and cervical TDR. The clinical outcomes and the in-hospital costs (theater plus hospital stay plus implant) were similar between the plate plus autograft (£2920), plate plus cage plus bone substitute (£2530), cage only (£1930), and TDR groups (£2435). An Australian federal government report, however, found ACDF ($15,300 Australian dollars) to be less expensive than cervical TDR ($24,027 Australian dollars), while calculating the costs of hospitalization, prosthesis, and medical fees.[60]

Summary: ACDF Versus Cervical TDR

ACDF is associated with favorable clinical outcomes with respect to relief of neck and arm pain. The short-term results of TDR are equivalent or compare favorably with ACDF. In addition, the drawbacks of ACDF, such as like ALD and bone graft donor site morbidity, can potentially be obviated by TDR but longer-term follow-up is necessary to make definitive treatment recommendations. There seems to be considerable variation in the cost of ACDF and TDR across the globe.

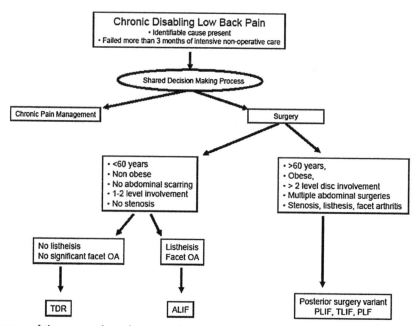

Fig. 1. A summary of the approach to the surgical management of chronic low back pain. ALIF, anterior lumbar interbody fusion; OA, osteoarthritis; PLF, posterolateral fusion; PLIF, posterior lumbar interbody fusion; TDR, total disk replacement; TLIF, transforaminal lumbar interbody fusion.

THE PHILOSOPHY

In the presence of the "refuse to fuse" group, the "I don't believe in disk replacement" group, and the extensively Internet-educated patients pulling in different directions, it can become a challenge for a voice of rationality to be heard. Based on evidence from literature, clinical experience, and a collaborative effort with patients, the authors practice a stepwise approach for the management of chronic degenerative low back pain (excluding spondylolisthesis and stenosis) and neck pain. Following a diagnostic work-up, patients undergo an intensive rehabilitation course consisting of structured physiotherapy that incorporates cognitive training and a psychologic assessment. Facet injections are performed as a diagnostic and therapeutic measure, being fully aware of its limitations. If there has been no improvement at the 3-month mark, patients are reassessed by the surgical team with input from physiotherapists. If there is no clinicoradiologic correlation and the patient continues to suffer from severe pain, pain pharmacotherapy is initiated. If a surgically treatable organic cause of the symptoms is elucidated, the patient is offered surgery based on a shared decision-making process. The approach to surgical decision making for one-level disk lumbar disorders is detailed in **Fig. 1**. The chart and approach is not valid for (1) two-level disk disease where one level exhibits advanced degeneration and the second level exhibits early stage degeneration, (2) postmicrodiskectomy states, (3) adjacent-level disk degeneration, and (4) degenerative disk disease with segmental coronal plane deformity or early lumbar degenerative scoliosis. A discussion on these conditions is outside the scope of this article.

A similar stepwise approach is followed while managing cervical degenerative conditions. Because cervical disk replacement is not funded by the Australian federal government at this stage, most eligible patients undergo an ACDF.

SUMMARY

In the absence of a magic wand to cure chronic degenerative axial spinal pain, a holistic approach incorporating a stepwise approach starting with nonoperative modalities (physiotherapy, spinal injections, pain counseling, and pharmacotherapy) is advisable. Surgery in the form of either spinal fusion of TDR should be reserved for recalcitrant cases. Although the short-term clinical outcomes following fusion and disk replacement are similar, TDR has the potential to reduce the incidence of ALD and obviate the complications associated with autologous bone graft.

REFERENCES

1. Frymoyer JW, Pope MH, Clements JH, et al. Risk factors in low-back pain: an epidemiological survey. J Bone Joint Surg Am 2009;1983(65):213–8.
2. Andersson GBJ. Epidemiological features of chronic low-back pain. Lancet 1999;354:581–5.
3. Rao R. Neck pain, cervical radiculopathy, and cervical myelopathy: pathophysiology, natural history, and clinical evaluation. J Bone Joint Surg Am 2002;84(10):1872–81.
4. Cote P, Cassidy JD, Carroll L. The Saskatchewan Health and Back Pain Survey. The prevalence of neck pain and related disability in Saskatchewan adults. Spine (Phila Pa 1976) 1998;23(15):1689–98.
5. Hart LG, Deyo RA, Cherkin DC. Physician office visits for low back pain: frequency, clinical evaluation, and treatment patterns from a US national survey. Spine 1995;20(1):11–9.
6. Hestbaek L, Leboeuf-Yde C, Manniche C. Low back pain: what is the long-term course? A review of studies of general patient populations. Eur Spine J 2003;12(2):149–65.
7. Dunn KM, Croft PR. Epidemiology and natural history of low back pain. Eura Medicophys 2004;40:9–13.
8. Pai S, Sundaram LJ. Low back pain: an economic assessment in the United States. Orthop Clin North Am 2004;35(1):1–5.
9. Ekman M, Jonhagen S, Hunsche E, et al. Burden of illness of chronic low back pain in Sweden: a cross-sectional, retrospective study in primary care setting. Spine (Phila Pa 1976) 2005;30(15):1777–85.
10. Walker BF, Muller R, Grant WD. Low back pain in Australian adults: the economic burden. Asia Pac J Public Health 2003;15(2):79–87.
11. Martin BI, Deyo RA, Mirza SK, et al. Expenditures and health status among adults with back and neck problems. JAMA 2008;299(6):656–64.
12. Brisby H. Pathology and possible mechanisms of nervous system response to disc degeneration. J Bone Joint Surg Am 2006;88(Suppl 2):68–71.
13. Kikuchi S. New concept for backache: biopsychosocial pain syndrome. Eur Spine J 2008;17(Suppl 4):421–7.
14. Huang RC, Lim MR, Girardi FP, et al. The prevalence of contraindications to total disc replacement in a cohort of lumbar surgical patients. Spine (Phila Pa 1976) 2004;29(22):2538–41.
15. Wong DA, Annesser B, Birney T, et al. Incidence of contraindications to total disc arthroplasty: a retrospective review of 100 consecutive fusion patients with a specific analysis of facet arthrosis. Spine J 2007;7(1):5–11.

16. Auerbach JD, Jones KJ, Fras CI, et al. The prevalence of indications and contraindications to cervical total disc replacement. Spine J 2008;8(5):711–6.

17. Albee F. Transplantation of a portion of the tibia into the spine for Pott's disease. JAMA 1911;57:885–6.

18. Hibbs RA. An operation for progressive spinal deformities. N Y Med J 1911;93:1013.

19. Deyo RA, Mirza SK. Trends and variations in the use of spine surgery. Clin Orthop Relat Res 2006;443:139–46.

20. Cook C, Santos GC, Lima R, et al. Geographic variation in lumbar fusion for degenerative disorders: 1990 to 2000. Spine J 2007;7(5):552–7.

21. Panjabi M, Henderson G, Abjornson C, et al. Multidirectional testing of one- and two-level ProDisc-L versus simulated fusions. Spine (Phila Pa 1976) 2007;32(12):1311–9.

22. Panjabi M, Malcolmson G, Teng E, et al. Hybrid testing of lumbar CHARITE discs versus fusions. Spine (Phila Pa 1976) 2007;32(9):959–66 [discussion: 967].

23. Ghiselli G, Wang JC, Bhatia NN, et al. Adjacent segment degeneration in the lumbar spine. J Bone Joint Surg Am 2004;86(7):1497–503.

24. Fenton JJ, Mirza SK, Lahad A, et al. Variation in reported safety of lumbar interbody fusion: influence of industrial sponsorship and other study characteristics. Spine (Phila Pa 1976) 2007;32(4):471–80.

25. Sasso RC, LeHuec JC, Shaffrey C. Iliac crest bone graft donor site pain after anterior lumbar interbody fusion: a prospective patient satisfaction outcome assessment. J Spinal Disord Tech 2005;18(Suppl):S77–81.

26. Gibson S, McLeod I, Wardlaw D, et al. Allograft versus autograft in instrumented posterolateral lumbar spinal fusion: a randomized control trial. Spine (Phila Pa 1976) 2002;27(15):1599–603.

27. Putzier M, Strube P, Funk JF, et al. Allogenic versus autologous cancellous bone in lumbar segmental spondylodesis: a randomized prospective study. Eur Spine J 2009;18(5):687–95.

28. Katayama Y, Matsuyama Y, Yoshihara H, et al. Clinical and radiographic outcomes of posterolateral lumbar spine fusion in humans using recombinant human bone morphogenetic protein-2: an average five-year follow-up study. Int Orthop 2009;33(4):1061–7.

29. Cahill KS, Chi JH, Day A, et al. Prevalence, complications, and hospital charges associated with use of bone-morphogenetic proteins in spinal fusion procedures. JAMA 2009;302(1):58–66.

30. Bono CM, Lee CK. The influence of subdiagnosis on radiographic and clinical outcomes after lumbar fusion for degenerative disc disorders: an analysis of the literature from two decades. Spine (Phila Pa 1976) 2005;30(2):227–34.

31. Buttermann GR, Garvey TA, Hunt AF, et al. Lumbar fusion results related to diagnosis. Spine (Phila Pa 1976) 1998;23(1):116–27.

32. Glassman SD, Carreon LY, Djurasovic M, et al. Lumbar fusion outcomes stratified by specific diagnostic indication. Spine J 2009;9(1):13–21.

33. Slosar PJ, Reynolds JB, Schofferman J, et al. Patient satisfaction after circumferential lumbar fusion. Spine (Phila Pa 1976) 2000;25(6):722–6.

34. Christensen FB. Lumbar spinal fusion: outcome in relation to surgical methods, choice of implant and postoperative rehabilitation. Acta Orthop Scand Suppl 2004;75(313):2–43.

35. Soegaard R, Bunger CE, Christiansen T, et al. Circumferential fusion is dominant over posterolateral fusion in a long-term perspective: cost-utility evaluation of a randomized controlled trial in severe, chronic low back pain. Spine (Phila Pa 1976) 2007;32(22):2405–14.

36. Christensen FB, Hansen ES, Eiskjaer SP, et al. Circumferential lumbar spinal fusion with Brantigan cage versus posterolateral fusion with titanium Cotrel-Dubousset instrumentation: a prospective, randomized clinical study of 146 patients. Spine (Phila Pa 1976) 2002;27(23):2674–83.

37. Videbaek TS, Christensen FB, Soegaard R, et al. Circumferential fusion improves outcome in comparison with instrumented posterolateral fusion: long-term results of a randomized clinical trial. Spine (Phila Pa 1976) 2006;31(25):2875–80.

38. Fritzell P, Hagg O, Wessberg P, et al. Chronic low back pain and fusion: a comparison of three surgical techniques: a prospective multicenter randomized study from the Swedish lumbar spine study group. Spine (Phila Pa 1976) 2002;27(11):1131–41.

39. Han X, Zhu Y, Cui C, et al. A meta-analysis of circumferential fusion versus instrumented posterolateral fusion in the lumbar spine. Spine 2009;34(17):E618–25.

40. Fairbank J, Frost H, Wilson-MacDonald J, et al. Randomised controlled trial to compare surgical stabilisation of the lumbar spine with an intensive rehabilitation programme for patients with chronic low back pain: the MRC spine stabilisation trial. BMJ 2005;330(7502):1233.

41. Brox JI, Reikeras O, Nygaard O, et al. Lumbar instrumented fusion compared with cognitive intervention and exercises in patients with chronic back pain after previous surgery for disc herniation: a prospective randomized controlled study. Pain 2006;122(1–2):145–55.

42. Brox JI, Sorensen R, Friis A, et al. Randomized clinical trial of lumbar instrumented fusion and cognitive intervention and exercises in patients with chronic low back pain and disc degeneration. Spine (Phila Pa 1976) 2003;28(17):1913–21.

43. Fritzell P, Hagg O, Wessberg P, et al. 2001 Volvo Award Winner in Clinical Studies: Lumbar fusion versus nonsurgical treatment for chronic low back pain: a multicenter randomized controlled trial from

the Swedish Lumbar Spine Study Group. Spine (Phila Pa 1976) 2001;26(23):2521–32 [discussion: 2532–4].

44. Resnick DK, Choudhri TF, Dailey AT, et al. Guidelines for the performance of fusion procedures for degenerative disease of the lumbar spine. Part 7: intractable low-back pain without stenosis or spondylolisthesis. J Neurosurg Spine 2005; 2(6):670–2.

45. Mirza SK, Deyo RA. Systematic review of randomized trials comparing lumbar fusion surgery to nonoperative care for treatment of chronic back pain. Spine (Phila Pa 1976) 2007;32(7):816–23.

46. Chou R, Baisden J, Carragee EJ, et al. Surgery for low back pain: a review of the evidence for an American Pain Society Clinical Practice Guideline. Spine (Phila Pa 1976) 2009;34(10):1094–109.

47. Ibrahim T, Tleyjeh IM, Gabbar O. Surgical versus non-surgical treatment of chronic low back pain: a meta-analysis of randomised trials. Int Orthop 2008;32(1):107–13.

48. Szpalski M, Gunzburg R, Mayer M. Spine arthroplasty: a historical review. Eur Spine J 2002; 11(Suppl 2):S65–84.

49. Huang RC, Tropiano P, Marnay T, et al. Range of motion and adjacent level degeneration after lumbar total disc replacement. Spine J 2006;6(3):242–7.

50. Lemaire JP, Carrier H, Sariali el-H, et al. Clinical and radiological outcomes with the Charite artificial disc: a 10-year minimum follow-up. J Spinal Disord Tech 2005;18(4):353–9.

51. David T. Long-term results of one-level lumbar arthroplasty: minimum 10-year follow-up of the CHARITE artificial disc in 106 patients. Spine (Phila Pa 1976) 2007;32(6):661–6.

52. Blumenthal S, McAfee PC, Guyer RD, et al. A prospective, randomized, multicenter Food and Drug Administration investigational device exemptions study of lumbar total disc replacement with the CHARITE artificial disc versus lumbar fusion: part I: evaluation of clinical outcomes. Spine (Phila Pa 1976) 2005;30(14):1565–75 [discussion: E1387–591].

53. Guyer RD, McAfee PC, Banco RJ, et al. Prospective, randomized, multicenter Food and Drug Administration investigational device exemption study of lumbar total disc replacement with the CHARITE artificial disc versus lumbar fusion: five-year follow-up. Spine J 2009;9(5):374–86.

54. Tropiano P, Huang RC, Girardi FP, et al. Lumbar total disc replacement: seven to eleven-year follow-up. J Bone Joint Surg Am 2005;87(3):490–6.

55. Zigler J, Delamarter R, Spivak JM, et al. Results of the prospective, randomized, multicenter Food and Drug Administration investigational device exemption study of the ProDisc-L total disc replacement versus circumferential fusion for the treatment of 1-level degenerative disc disease. Spine (Phila Pa 1976) 2007;32(11):1155–62 [discussion: 1163].

56. Shim CS, Lee SH, Shin HD, et al. CHARITE versus ProDisc: a comparative study of a minimum 3-year follow-up. Spine (Phila Pa 1976) 2007;32(9):1012–8.

57. Guyer RD, Tromanhauser SG, Regan JJ. An economic model of one-level lumbar arthroplasty versus fusion. Spine J 2007;7(5):558–62.

58. Patel VV, Estes S, Lindley EM, et al. Lumbar spinal fusion versus anterior lumbar disc replacement: the financial implications. J Spinal Disord Tech 2008;21(7):473–6.

59. Levin DA, Bendo JA, Quirno M, et al. Comparative charge analysis of one- and two-level lumbar total disc arthroplasty versus circumferential lumbar fusion. Spine (Phila Pa 1976) 2007;32(25):2905–9.

60. Artificial intervertebral disc replacement (total disc arthroplasty). Medical Services Advisory Committee - Assessment Report. 2006. Available at: http://www.msac.gov.au/internet/msac/publishing.nsf/Content/2CDBC3816FDE8D20CA2575AD0082FD8E/%24File/1090%20-%20Artificial%20intervertebral%20disc%20replacement%20Report.pdf. Accessed November 15, 2009.

61. Anderson PA, Puschak TJ, Sasso RC. Comparison of short-term SF-36 results between total joint arthroplasty and cervical spine decompression and fusion or arthroplasty. Spine (Phila Pa 1976) 2009;34(2): 176–83.

62. DiAngelo DJ, Roberston JT, Metcalf NH, et al. Biomechanical testing of an artificial cervical joint and an anterior cervical plate. J Spinal Disord Tech 2003;16(4):314–23.

63. Eck JC, Humphreys SC, Lim TH, et al. A biomechanical study on the effect of cervical spine fusion on adjacent-level intradiscal pressure and segmental motion. Spine (Phila Pa 1976) 2002;27(22):2431–4.

64. Chang UK, Kim DH, Lee MC, et al. Changes in adjacent-level disc pressure and facet joint force after cervical arthroplasty compared with cervical discectomy and fusion. J Neurosurg Spine 2007; 7(1):33–9.

65. Goffin J, Geusens E, Vantomme N, et al. Long-term follow-up after interbody fusion of the cervical spine. J Spinal Disord Tech 2004;17(2):79–85.

66. Hilibrand AS, Carlson GD, Palumbo MA, et al. Radiculopathy and myelopathy at segments adjacent to the site of a previous anterior cervical arthrodesis. J Bone Joint Surg Am 1999;81(4):519–28.

67. Henderson CM, Hennessy RG, Shuey HM Jr, et al. Posterior-lateral foraminotomy as an exclusive operative technique for cervical radiculopathy: a review of 846 consecutively operated cases. Neurosurgery 1983;13(5):504–12.

68. Robertson JT, Papadopoulos SM, Traynelis VC. Assessment of adjacent-segment disease in patients treated with cervical fusion or

arthroplasty: a prospective 2-year study. J Neurosurg Spine 2005;3(6):417–23.

69. Iseda T, Goya T, Nakano S, et al. Serial changes in signal intensities of the adjacent discs on T2-weighted sagittal images after surgical treatment of cervical spondylosis: anterior interbody fusion versus expansive laminoplasty. Acta Neurochir (Wien) 2001;143(7):707–10.

70. Phillips FM, Tzermiadianos MN, Voronov LI, et al. Effect of two-level total disc replacement on cervical spine kinematics. Spine (Phila Pa 1976) 2009; 34(22):E794–9.

71. Sasso RC, Smucker JD, Hacker RJ, et al. Artificial disc versus fusion: a prospective, randomized study with 2-year follow-up on 99 patients. Spine (Phila Pa 1976) 2007;32(26):2933–40 [discussion: 2941–2].

72. Sasso RC, Smucker JD, Hacker RJ, et al. Clinical outcomes of BRYAN cervical disc arthroplasty: a prospective, randomized, controlled, multicenter trial with 24-month follow-up. J Spinal Disord Tech 2007;20(7):481–91.

73. Coric D, Finger F, Boltes P. Prospective randomized controlled study of the Bryan Cervical Disc: early clinical results from a single investigational site. J Neurosurg Spine 2006;4(1):31–5.

74. Heller JG, Sasso RC, Papadopoulos SM, et al. Comparison of BRYAN cervical disc arthroplasty with anterior cervical decompression and fusion: clinical and radiographic results of a randomized, controlled, clinical trial. Spine (Phila Pa 1976) 2009;34(2):101–7.

75. Cheng L, Nie L, Zhang L, et al. Fusion versus Bryan Cervical Disc in two-level cervical disc disease: a prospective, randomised study. Int Orthop 2009; 33(5):1347–51.

76. Nabhan A, Ahlhelm F, Shariat K, et al. The ProDisc-C prosthesis: clinical and radiological experience 1 year after surgery. Spine (Phila Pa 1976) 2007; 32(18):1935–41.

77. Nabhan A, Ahlhelm F, Pitzen T, et al. Disc replacement using Pro-Disc C versus fusion: a prospective randomised and controlled radiographic and clinical study. Eur Spine J 2007;16(3):423–30.

78. Murrey D, Janssen M, Delamarter R, et al. Results of the prospective, randomized, controlled multicenter Food and Drug Administration investigational device exemption study of the ProDisc-C total disc replacement versus anterior discectomy and fusion for the treatment of 1-level symptomatic cervical disc disease. Spine J 2009;9(4):275–86.

79. Bhadra AK, Raman AS, Casey AT, et al. Single-level cervical radiculopathy: clinical outcome and cost-effectiveness of four techniques of anterior cervical discectomy and fusion and disc arthroplasty. Eur Spine J 2009;18(2):232–7.

80. Gibson JA, Waddell G. Surgery for degenerative lumbar spondylosis. Cochrane Database Syst Rev 2005;(4):CD001352. DOI: 10.1002/14651858. CD001352.pub3. Accessed November 15, 2009.

81. Carreon LY, Glassman SD, Howard J. Fusion and nonsurgical treatment for symptomatic lumbar degenerative disease: a systematic review of Oswestry Disability Index and MOS Short Form-36 outcomes. Spine J 2008;8(5):747–55.

82. Berg S, Tullberg T, Branth B, et al. Total disc replacement compared to lumbar fusion: a randomised controlled trial with 2-year follow-up. Eur Spine J 2009;18(10):1512–9.

83. Anderson PA, Sasso RC, Rouleau JP, et al. The Bryan Cervical Disc: wear properties and early clinical results. Spine J 2004;4(6 Suppl):303S–9S.

84. Heidecke V, Burkert W, Brucke M, et al. Intervertebral disc replacement for cervical degenerative disease: clinical results and functional outcome at two years in patients implanted with the Bryan Cervical Disc prosthesis. Acta Neurochir (Wien) 2008;150(5):453–9 [discussion: 459].

85. Mummaneni PV, Burkus JK, Haid RW, et al. Clinical and radiographic analysis of cervical disc arthroplasty compared with allograft fusion: a randomized controlled clinical trial. J Neurosurg Spine 2007;6(3): 198–209.

86. Beaurain J, Bernard P, Dufour T, et al. Intermediate clinical and radiological results of cervical TDR (Mobi-C) with up to 2 years of follow-up. Eur Spine J 2009;18(6):841–50.

87. Park JH, Roh KH, Cho JY, et al. Comparative analysis of cervical arthroplasty using mobi-c(r) and anterior cervical discectomy and fusion using the Solis(r) -Cage. J Korean Neurosurg Soc 2008; 44(4):217–21.

88. Pimenta L, McAfee PC, Cappuccino A, et al. Superiority of multilevel cervical arthroplasty outcomes versus single-level outcomes: 229 consecutive PCM prostheses. Spine (Phila Pa 1976) 2007; 32(12):1337–44.

Contemporary Management of Symptomatic Lumbar Spinal Stenosis

Mladen Djurasovic, MD*, Steven D. Glassman, MD,
Leah Y. Carreon, MD, MSc, John R. Dimar II, MD

KEYWORDS

- Lumbar spinal stenosis • Laminectomy
- Conservative care • Randomized trials

Lumbar spinal stenosis is a common cause of impaired quality of life and diminished functional capacity in the elderly.[1] With the aging of the United States population, lumbar stenosis will be increasingly diagnosed and treated by primary care physicians and surgical and nonsurgical specialists alike. Because of the advance of noninvasive imaging modalities, spinal stenosis is becoming more frequently identified, and has become the most frequent cause for spinal surgery in patients older than 65 years.[2,3] The rate of spinal surgery in the Medicare population has increased by 57%, from 2.1 to 3.4 per 1000, between 1988 and 1997, but in addition it has shown tremendous regional variation, both nationally and internationally.[4]

Despite the ubiquitous nature of this condition, considerable controversy exists regarding the preferred treatment, and many commonly used treatments lack high-level evidence regarding their efficacy. A Cochrane database review in 2005 noted that most published articles consisted of uncontrolled case series or prospective cohort studies, and the few randomized trials that have been reported were performed on a small number of patients and reported mixed surgical indications.[5] The current emphasis that is being placed on comparative effectiveness and evidence-based clinical practice has highlighted the need for high-quality data to help guide the treatment of lumbar stenosis patients. In particular, level I evidence comparing the effectiveness of surgical and nonsurgical treatment has been lacking. Recent studies, such as the Spine Patient Outcomes Research Trial (SPORT), have addressed some of these deficiencies and are discussed in this article.

PATHOPHYSIOLOGY AND CLINICAL PRESENTATION

Spinal stenosis can be broadly classified as congenital or acquired (degenerative).[6] Congenital lumbar spinal stenosis is rare, and is caused by a congenital narrowing of the spinal canal, mostly resulting from short pedicles.[7,8] The anatomic changes responsible for degenerative lumbar spinal stenosis show considerable overlap with those that are seen during the normal aging of the lumbar spinal motion segment. Degeneration is believed to begin in the intervertebral disk where biochemical changes such as cell death and loss of proteoglycan and water content lead to progressive disk bulging and collapse. This process leads to an increased stress transfer to the posterior facet joints, which accelerates cartilaginous degeneration, hypertrophy, and osteophyte formation; this is associated with thickening and buckling of the ligamentum flavum. The combination of the ventral disk bulging and osteophyte formation and the

Norton Leatherman Spine Center, 210 East Gray Street, Suite 900, Louisville, KY 40202, USA
* Corresponding author.
E-mail address: djuraso@hotmail.com

Orthop Clin N Am 41 (2010) 183–191
doi:10.1016/j.ocl.2009.12.003
0030-5898/10/$ – see front matter © 2010 Elsevier Inc. All rights reserved.

dorsal facet and ligamentum flavum hyptertrophy combine to circumferentially narrow the spinal canal and the space available for the neural elements.[8–12] This compression of the nerve roots of the cauda equina leads to the characteristic clinical signs and symptoms of lumbar spinal stenosis.

Patients with degenerative spinal stenosis are usually older than 40 years, and present with some combination of back and leg pain. The most specific presentation of lumbar spinal stenosis is neurogenic claudication.[13] Patients develop a burning or aching pain in the lumbar region, buttocks, or lower extremities when in upright posture, and these are often associated with numbness, paresthesias, or subjective weakness. Typically their symptoms are worsened by the extension of the spine, which exacerbates the pathologic narrowing of the spinal canal. Patients report that standing, walking, and climbing stairs will cause symptoms to develop, and that these symptoms can be partially relieved by flexion of the spine, such as sitting or leaning forward (eg, pushing a shopping cart). Impaired walking ability is often an important factor in causing these patients to seek treatment. Neurogenic claudication symptoms must be distinguished from vascular claudication, which can mimic spinal stenosis. Although neurogenic claudication is the most characteristic presentation of lumbar spinal stenosis, not all patients will exhibit this constellation of symptoms. Many will report unilateral or bilateral radicular symptoms rather than true claudication. Neurologic findings on physical examination are unusual, and the diagnosis is generally made based on characteristic subjective complaints coupled with radiographic evidence of spinal canal narrowing from magnetic resonance imaging (MRI), computed tomography (CT), or CT myelography.

NONSURGICAL TREATMENT

Although the role of surgery has certainly been debated in the treatment of lumbar spinal stenosis, little high-level evidence is available to recommend specific nonsurgical treatments. In 1987, the Quebec Task Force on Spinal Disorders concluded that no large-sample, randomized controlled trials were available regarding specific conservative treatments for lumbar spinal stenosis.[14] Current nonsurgical treatment largely follows established practice patterns, empiric evidence, and expert opinion.[13] As the symptoms of lumbar stenosis are slowly evolving, a trial of conservative treatment is generally recommended. Commonly used conservative treatments for lumbar spinal stenosis include activity modification, medications, physical therapy, home exercise therapy, and spinal injections.[15]

Activity modification generally consists of the avoidance of those activities that place mechanical stress on the lower back, particularly those that place the spine in extension, as this tends to exacerbate the symptoms. Although high-level evidence is lacking for the direct benefit of physical therapy or exercise for spinal stenosis,[16] most clinicians believe that a program of core strengthening exercise and aerobic conditioning can be of benefit in maintaining functional independence in these patients. Aerobic activities that maintain the spine in a slightly flexed posture, such as recumbent stationary bicycles or elliptical trainers, may be better tolerated by stenosis patients.

Nonsteroidal anti-inflammatory drugs (NSAIDs) are amongst the most commonly used medications for degenerative spinal conditions, particularly acute low back pain. Data demonstrating their efficacy in the long-term treatment of spinal stenosis is lacking.[17] These medications must be used with caution in the elderly because of side effects such as gastrointestinal bleeding or renal insufficiency. Routine screening of renal function is necessary if these drugs are to be used long-term. Similarly, muscle relaxants, which are commonly used in acute low back pain, should have a limited role in the long-term treatment of stenosis. Opioid analgesics have numerous long-term side effects including sedation, constipation, and the potential for dependency. Their use should be limited to controlling acute exacerbations of pain.

Epidural steroid injections (ESIs) may be beneficial in relieving radicular lower extremity symptoms in lumbar spinal stenosis. However, their use remains controversial and evidence regarding their effectiveness is conflicting. Cuckler and associates,[18] in a randomized controlled trial, found no short-term or long-term benefit of epidural injection of methylprednisolone with local anesthetic compared with an injection of saline and local anesthetic. Hoogmartens and Morelle,[19] in a retrospective review of 49 patients with lumbar spinal stenosis treated with epidural steroids, found that only 32% had acceptable pain relief at 2 years. In contrast, Riew and colleagues,[20] in a double-blind, prospective randomized trial, found that 71% of surgical candidates injected with a combination of betamethasone and bupivacaine were able to avoid surgery at 13-month follow-up, as compared with 33% of the patients who received bupivacaine alone. This benefit seemed to be maintained at 5-year follow-up.[21] In general, the limited use of ESI for exacerbations of symptoms are fairly well accepted by clinicians, but few data support the long-term benefit of multiple ESIs over prolonged periods. Their exact role in the treatment of lumbar spinal stenosis awaits further prospective study.

SURGICAL TREATMENT

The exact surgical procedure that needs to be performed depends on the exact pathoanatomy of the canal narrowing seen in any given patient. Stenosis can be anatomically classified as central stenosis, lateral recess stenosis, and foraminal stenosis.[15] Central stenosis is the narrowing of the central spinal canal from one edge of the dural tube to the other. Central stenosis most commonly occurs from a disk bulge anteriorly, or hypertrophied or infolded ligamentum flavum, or hypertrophic inferior articular facet posteriorly. Lateral recess stenosis is narrowing in the subarticular recess, bounded by the takeoff of the nerve root from the dural tube to the medial border of the pedicle. Lateral recess stenosis is most commonly caused by hypertrophy of the superior articular facet or the lateral insertion of the ligamentum flavum where it merges with the articular facet capsule. Again, an anteriorly bulging disk can contribute to lateral recess stenosis. Foraminal spinal stenosis occurs in the neuroforamen itself, bounded by the disk and vertebral endplate margins anteriorly, the pars interarticularis posteriorly, and the pedicles superiorly and inferiorly. Compression of the nerve root in the neuroforamen is most commonly caused by a combination of a bulging disk and rostral-caudal collapse of the pedicles due to disk degeneration and collapse. Compression of the neural elements can occur in one or several of the anatomic zones.

Standard surgical treatment of lumbar spinal stenosis consists of a decompressive lumbar laminectomy.[12] Laminectomy begins with removal of the respective spinous process and supraspinous and interspinous ligaments to gain access to the interlaminar space in the midline. The lamina is then thinned with a rongeur or high-speed drill followed by removal using various Kerrison rongeurs. Removal of the hypertrophic ligamentum flavum then follows. The ligamentum flavum is carefully detached from the leading edge of the lamina below and from the undersurface of the lamina above. It is then removed using Kerrison rongeurs. The removal of lamina and ligamentum is carried laterally out to the level of the lateral recess, where the medial border of the pedicle can be palpated from within the canal using a curved ball-tipped probe. A partial medial facetectomy is then performed. The medial one-third to half of the facet

is removed using 45°-angled Kerrison rongeurs. Finally, decompression of the nerve root in the neuroforamen can be performed with small (eg, 2 mm) Kerrison rongeurs. On completion of the decompression, a 3- to 4-mm curved ball-tipped probe should pass easily into the subarticular recess and then the neuroforamen, following the course of the nerve root as it exits the spinal canal. If the area of compression is more limited on preoperative imaging studies, a more limited procedure such as a unilateral partial laminotomy and foraminotomy can be performed.

Two surgical techniques that deserve mention at this point are spinal fusion and interspinous process devices. The indications to perform spinal fusion in combination with laminectomy are controversial and are beyond the scope of this article. In general, spinal fusion is indicated in situations whereby spinal instability is preexisting at the time of surgical decompression and decompression is likely to make instability worse, or in situations whereby the decompressive procedure is likely to induce postoperative instability. Interspinous process devices (eg, X-STOP [Kyphon Inc, Sunnyvale, CA, USA], Wallis [Abbott Spine Inc, Austin, TX, USA], or DIAM [Medtronic Sofamor Danek Inc, Memphis, TN, USA]), have recently emerged as an alternative to decompressive procedures such as laminectomy. These devices are designed to act as a block to hypertension posteriorly at the level of the facet, to prevent exacerbation of canal narrowing during extension postures of the spine. A recent prospective randomized trial suggests that the use of one of these devices is superior to conservative care in the treatment of symptomatic lumbar spinal stenosis.[22] Interspinous process devices are a promising technology in the treatment of lumbar spinal stenosis, but their exact indications and role in the treatment of stenosis remain to be seen.

EVIDENCE FOR SURGICAL TREATMENT OF SPINAL STENOSIS

The literature regarding the surgical treatment of lumbar spinal stenosis has shown an evolution from uncontrolled case series to prospective randomized trials comparing surgical with nonoperative treatment (ie, SPORT). Several of these studies are outlined in **Table 1**. Their side-by-side comparison is not designed to directly compare the merits of one study to another, but is meant to illustrate the evolution and natural progression of the literature associated with surgical treatment of spinal stenosis.

Verbiest[23] first described the pathoanatomy, clinical presentation, and radiographic findings of

Table 1
Evidentiary table: a summary of quality of evidence supporting surgical decompression for lumbar spinal stenosis

References	Study Design	Main Findings	Strengths	Weaknesses	Level of Evidence
Verbiest[24] J Bone Joint J Surg, 1977	Retrospective case series	Two-thirds experience relief	Early case series	Study design; Subjective grading criteria	IV
Johnsson et al[33] Spine, 1991	Retrospective cohort and natural history study	70% patients remain stable; 15% improve; 15% deteriorate	First report of natural history	Retrospective design; Limited sample size	IV
Katz et al[34,35] J Bone Joint Surg, 1991 Spine, 1996	Retrospective case series	57% success; Clinical results deteriorate with time	Long-term follow-up; Patient-focused outcomes measures	Retrospective design; Many spondylolisthesis pts not fused	IV
Herno et al[36] Spine, 1993	Retrospective case series	69% good-to-excellent long-term; No deterioration with time	Standard outcomes measures (ODI); Long-term follow-up	Retrospective design; No baseline outcomes measures	IV
Airaksinen et al[37] Spine, 1997	Retrospective case series	62% clinical success; Average. 4 y ODI = 34 pts; Severe stenosis did better	Large sample size; Standard outcomes measures	Retrospective design; No baseline outcomes measures	IV
Cornefjord et al[38] Eur Spine J, 2000	Retrospective case series	65% patient satisfaction; Fusion patients simulate outcomes to unfused	Long-term follow-up	Retrospective; Mixed patient group; No baseline outcomes	IV
Jönsson et al[39] Spine, 1997	Prospective cohort study	67% excellent results at 2 y; 52% at 5 y	Prospective design; Consecutive pts; Large sample size	Lack of control group; No standardized outcomes measures	II
Atlas et al[40-42] Spine, 1996, 2000, 2005	Prospective observational (nonrandomized) study	Improvement in 55% of surgical patients, 28% of conservative at 1 y	Prospective; Standard outcomes (Roland-Morris, SF-36)	Nonrandomized	II
Amundsen et al[43] Spine, 2000	Prospective, Partial randomization	Randomized group 92% excellent or fair with surgery	Prospective; Long-term follow-up	No standard outcomes measures; Only 31/100 patients randomized; Selection bias	II

Mariconda et al[44] J Spinal Disord, 2002	Prospective, partial randomization	Unilateral laminectomy At 4 y, 68% good-to-excellent in surgical vs 33% conservative	Prospective Partial randomization	Small sample size No standard outcomes measures	II
Athiviraham & Yen[45] Clin Orthop Relat Res, 2007	Prospective, observational (nonrandomized) study	62% better with surgery 25% with conservative care	Prospective Standardized outcomes measures (Roland-Morris)	Nonrandomized Mixed patient population (fusions)	II
Malmivaara et al[46] Spine, 2007	Prospective randomized, controlled trial	Surgical pts superior to conservative at 2 y (ODI, LBP, leg pain)	Prospective randomized Standard measures (ODI) Strict inclusion criteria	Mixed patient population (fusions) Limited sample size	I
Weinstein et al[47] N Engl J Med, 2008	Prospective, randomized controlled trial	As-treated analysis: surgical treatment superior to conservative at 2 y	Prospective RCT Standard measures Large sample size	High crossover Limited follow-up	I

Abbreviations: LBP, low back pain; ODI, Oswestry Disability Index; pts, patients; RCT, randomized controlled trial; SF-36, 36-item Short-Form General Health Survey.

lumbar spinal stenosis in his landmark report in 1954. He published his results of the surgical treatment of 147 patients in 1977[24] and noted that approximately two-thirds reported relief of their sciatica or intermittent claudication, but lumbago often persisted. Several other case series of the surgical treatment of lumbar stenosis were published in the 1970s and 1980s[25–31] with similar success rates based on subjective surgeon assessment, before studies with more standardized assessment techniques began to emerge in the 1990s.

Johnsson and colleagues[32] made an important contribution to the stenosis literature in 1992 by describing the natural history of the disease. Previous studies rarely reported on the clinical course of patients with stenosis who were treated with observation, and many surgeons held to the belief that the natural history was poor. Johnsson followed 32 patients for an average 4 years of follow-up and showed that, based on subjective visual analog scores, 70% of patients reported no significant change in symptoms, 15% showed significant improvement, whereas 15% showed some deterioration. No severe deterioration was seen in any patient. In a separate report, Johnsson and colleagues[33] retrospectively compared the results of 44 patients who were surgically treated for stenosis and 16 unmatched patients treated nonoperatively. At 3- to 5-year follow-up, 60% of surgically treated patients reported a feeling of improvement, compared with 33% of conservatively treated patients. The investigators concluded that observation is a reasonable treatment option for lumbar stenosis and that significant neurologic deterioration is rare.

Katz and colleagues[34] published 2 reports, which suggested that previously published success rates may overestimate the success of lumbar laminectomy and that the results may deteriorate over time. These investigators retrospectively studied 88 patients, all of whom underwent lumbar laminectomy from 1983 to 1986 by a single surgeon. At average 4-year follow-up, 57% had acceptable clinical results; 30% reported severe residual pain, and 46% still could not walk 2 blocks. The investigators identified coexisting illnesses, especially lower extremity comorbidities such as hip or knee osteoarthritis, as the strongest risk factor for poor clinical outcomes. A subsequent study of the same cohort at 8-year follow-up[35] showed that 23% required reoperation, 33% reported severe back pain, and more than 80% still had significant limitations in walking ability. Despite these disappointing objective results, 75% of the patients were subjectively satisfied with their surgery and 82% would undergo the operation again if they could go back in time. Twenty-two patients had a preoperative spondylolisthesis, and only 8 of these 22 underwent surgery for concomitant fusion.

Several other retrospective studies with larger patient sample sizes and more objective clinical outcomes criteria were published in the 1990s. Herno and colleagues[36] specifically examined whether clinical results of laminectomy deteriorated over time. These investigators followed a cohort of 119 patients who underwent laminectomy and showed that between the seventh and the thirteenth year of follow-up, the average Oswestry Disability Index (ODI) score actually improved from 34.5 to 30.2, suggesting no significant deterioration over long-term follow-up. Airaksinen and colleagues[37] reported the largest series to date of lumbar laminectomy patients in 1997 (438 patients) and found an overall success rate of 62% at 4.3-year follow-up. This study found that preoperative diabetes, hip arthrosis, or prior spinal fracture predicted poor results, whereas more severe radiographic stenosis predicted better clinical outcomes. Cornefjord and colleagues[38] published results at 7-year follow-up again showing 65% subjective patient satisfaction, although this report included 61% of patients undergoing simultaneous arthrodesis. Walking ability was improved in most patients, with 64% being able to walk more than 1 km at follow-up. Jönsson and colleagues[39] performed the first prospective cohort study by following 105 patients undergoing laminectomy and evaluating their results at 4 months, 2 years, and 5 years after the surgery. These investigators found excellent results in 63%, 67%, and 52% of the patients at these time points, noting some deterioration of results with time. The reoperation rate of 18% at 5 years was similar to the findings reported by Katz and colleagues.[34]

In the current decade, studies have begun to directly compare the results of surgical treatment with nonoperative care. The Maine Lumbar Spine Study was a prospective observational cohort study of 81 patients treated surgically with laminectomy and 67 patients who were treated with the usual conservative care. Atlas and colleagues[40–42] published results of these patients in 3 separate reports at 1-year, 4-year and 8- to 10-year follow-up. Atlas' group found the predominant symptom of back or leg pain to be significantly improved in 55% of surgically treated patients at 1 year compared with 28% of nonsurgically treated patients. The study used standardized health-related quality of life measures and found that the Roland-Morris score and the 36-item Short-Form General Health Survey (SF-36) score were also superior in the surgically treated group, even after controlling for baseline difference in disability in the 2 groups. The relative superiority of surgical treatment diminished somewhat between the 4- and 10-year time points, but at 10 years, surgically treated patients still reported better leg pain scores and back-specific functional status. Amundsen and colleagues,[43] Mariconda and colleagues,[44] and Athiviraham and Yen[45] all published prospective, nonrandomized or partially randomized studies that showed superior outcomes of surgically treated patients compared with conservatively treated patients.

Malmivaara and colleagues[46] published the results of the first randomized controlled trial comparing surgical and conservative treatment for spinal stenosis. Fifty patients were randomized to surgical treatment and 44 patients to nonsurgical treatment. The investigators compared improvements in ODI, back pain and leg pain intensity, and walking ability at regular intervals of 2 years. ODI, back pain, and leg pain improvements were greater in the surgically treated patients, although walking ability did not differ between the 2 groups. The surgical group was mixed and included 10 instrumented posterolateral fusions. This study provided the only level I evidence for surgical treatment of spinal stenosis before the SPORT trial, which is described in the following section.

THE SPORT STUDY

The SPORT study[47] represents a significant step forward in evaluating common surgical treatments for the lumbar spine. The SPORT study was conceived as an effort to evaluate the effectiveness of surgical versus nonsurgical care for 3 of the most common surgically treated conditions of the lumbar spine, namely intervertebral disk herniation, spinal stenosis, and degenerative spondylolisthesis.[48] SPORT was a prospective, multicenter study, funded by the National Institute of Arthritis and Musculoskeletal and Skin Diseases (NIAMS) and the National Institutes of Health (NIH). The study was conducted at 13 multidisciplinary spine centers in 11 states with the Dartmouth Medical School (Dartmouth-Hitchcock Medical Center) serving as the coordinating center. SPORT actually consisted of 3 separate concurrent prospective trials for intervertebral disk herniation, lumbar spinal stenosis, and degenerative spondylolisthesis. The authors focus on the spinal stenosis study in the current discussion.

A unique design feature of SPORT was that patients who were eligible for the trial but who did not consent to randomization were enrolled in an observational cohort, in which the patient chose the treatment (surgical vs nonsurgical), but were otherwise followed in exactly the same manner as the randomized patients. A significant drawback of randomized trials for surgical treatments is the potential for the patient sample to differ from average patients treated for the same condition. The inclusion of an observational cohort allowed the investigators to test whether there were systematic differences in the type and severity of illness for patients who consented to randomization. This method allows some conclusions to be drawn about the generalizability of the findings of the study and also allows for combination of the randomized and observational arms of the trial in an "as-treated" analysis, thus increasing the sample size and statistical power of the study.[48]

Inclusion criteria for the spinal stenosis study included symptoms of neurogenic claudication or radiculopathy for at least 12 weeks, with confirmatory radiographic studies (MRI, CT), and overall patient health. These criteria were sufficient for a person to be considered a surgical candidate. Exclusion criteria included radiographic instability (spondylolisthesis, or 4-mm translational or 10° angular motion with flexion-extension radiographs), progressive neurologic deficit, poor overall health precluding surgical treatment, pregnancy, malignancy, fracture deformity, and a history of previous surgery. Using these criteria, 1091 patients were identified as being eligible for the study and 654 patients were successfully enrolled. Two hundred and eighty-nine patients were enrolled in the randomized cohort and 365 were enrolled in the observational cohort.

Of the 289 patients in the randomized arm of the study, 138 were randomized to surgical treatment and 151 to nonsurgical treatment. Surgical treatment consisted of a standard posterior laminectomy. Nonsurgical treatment was the usual care, and consisted of a minimum of active physical therapy, education, counseling with home exercise therapy, and NSAIDs. However, a standardized protocol was not imposed on the nonsurgical patients, and the physicians were free to prescribe other medications and interventions (eg, injection therapy) as deemed appropriate. Crossover and nonadherence were significant in the randomized arm of the study as only 67% of the patients who were randomized to surgery had actually undergone surgery by 2 years, and 43% of the patients who were initially randomized to nonoperative care actually had undergone surgery by the end of 2 years. In the observational cohort of 365 patients, 219 patients elected to have surgery and 146 patients chose nonsurgical care. Again, 22% of the nonsurgical patients in the observational cohort had surgery by the end of the 2-year follow-up period.

The investigators identified their primary outcome parameters a priori as the bodily pain and physical function subscales of the Medical Outcomes Study SF-36 as a measure of general health, and the modified ODI score as a measure of low back–specific disability. Secondary outcomes measures included patient-reported improvement, satisfaction with symptoms and care, and bothersomeness of stenosis and low back pain. Outcomes measures were collected at baseline, 6 weeks, 3 months, 6 months, 1 year, and 2 years. The primary analyses performed were the mean differences in improvement in outcomes measures between the surgical and nonsurgical groups at 2 years.

Study results were presented in an intent-to-treat as well as an as-treated analysis. Intent-to-treat analyses counted all patients based on which group they were randomized to at the beginning of the study, irrespective of which treatment they actually received. These methods are generally considered preferable as they minimize the potential for confounding baseline characteristics of the study groups. Thus, in the intent-to-treat analysis of SPORT, the nonsurgical group included 43% of patients who actually had undergone surgery. Obviously, in any study with such high crossover, the crossover patients will tend to bias the results toward the null hypothesis of no difference between treatments. Despite this very high crossover in the randomized cohort, surgical treatment was still superior to nonsurgical treatment in the bodily pain subscale of the SF-36 (7.8 patients, 95% confidence interval 1.5–14.1). Because of the high crossover, the investigators then presented an as-treated analysis in which the randomized and observational cohorts were combined, and patients were grouped according to the treatment that they actually received. A longitudinal regression model was created, which controlled for confounding baseline differences in the 2 groups. In this analysis, surgery was superior to nonsurgical treatment across all primary and secondary outcomes measures beginning at the 6-week time point and continuing on to 2 years. The investigators concluded that spinal stenosis patients treated with surgery showed greater improvements in pain, function, and satisfaction, as well as low back–specific and general health-related quality of life measures, than patients who were managed with nonoperative treatment.

SUMMARY

Spinal stenosis is a common degenerative condition affecting the lumbar spine in the elderly. Low back pain and leg pain, numbness, and subjective weakness cause significant disability in these patients, and their limited walking ability often leads them to seek treatment. With the continued aging of the population in United States, rising rates of spinal surgery, and limited societal resources to apply to medical care, the need for evidence-based treatment in spinal surgery has never been more acute. Recent studies have helped to clarify the role for surgery in the treatment of the spinal stenosis patient.

The symptoms of spinal stenosis are slowly evolving, and most patients can safely undergo a trial of conservative treatment. Many patients with mild to moderate symptoms can expect little change over time. Commonly used conservative care includes activity modification, medication, physical therapy or a home exercise program, and epidural cortisone injections. In patients with severe symptoms or in those who fail conservative care, surgical laminectomy will generally yield 60% to 70% successful results, which has been shown to be superior to continued conservative care. Some studies suggest some modest deterioration in surgical results over time, but subjective patient satisfaction seems to remain high. Future studies will hopefully clarify the role of arthrodesis and interspinous process devices. Effective communication and a shared decision-making process between the treating physician and patient will facilitate optimal outcomes for the patient with lumbar spinal stenosis.

REFERENCES

1. Lin SI, Lin RM, Huang LW. Disability in patients with degenerative lumbar spinal stenosis. Arch Phys Med Rehabil 2006;87:1250–6.
2. Deyo RA, Gray DT, Kreuter W, et al. United States trends in lumbar fusion surgery for degenerative conditions. Spine 2005;30:1441–5.
3. Weinstein JN, Lurie JD, Olson PR, et al. United States trends and regional variations in lumbar spine surgery: 1992–2003. Spine 2006;31:2707–14.
4. Cherkin DC, Deyo RA, Loser JD, et al. An international comparison of back surgery rates. Spine 1994;19:1201–6.
5. Gibson JN, Waddell G. Surgery for degenerative lumbar spondylosis. Cochrane Database Syst Rev 2005;(2):CD001352.
6. Arnoldi CC, Brodsky AE, Chauchoix J, et al. Lumbar spinal stenosis and nerve root entrapment syndromes: definition and classification. Clin Orthop Relat Res 1976;115:4–5.
7. Sarpyener MA. Congenital stricture of the spinal canal. J Bone Joint Surg Am 1945;27:70.
8. Verbiest H. Pathomorphologic aspects of developmental lumbar stenosis. Orthop Clin North Am 1975;6:177–96.
9. Buckwalter JA. Aging and degeneration of the human intervertebral disc. Spine 1995;20:1307–14.
10. Butler D, Trafimow JH, Anderson GB, et al. Discs degenerate before facets. Spine 1990;15:111–3.
11. Yong-Hing K, Reilly J, Kirkaldy-Willis WH. The ligamentum flavum. Spine 1976;1:226–34.
12. Dimar JR II, Djurasovic M, Carreon LY. Surgical management of degenerative spinal stenosis. Semin Spine Surg 2005;17:195–204.
13. Atlas SJ, Delitto A. Spinal stenosis: surgical versus nonsurgical treatment. Clin Orthop Relat Res 2006; 443:198–207.
14. Spitzer WO. Scientific approach to the assessment and management of activity-related spinal disorders. A monograph for clinicians. Report of the Quebec Task Force on Spinal Disorders. Spine 1987;12:S22–34.
15. Daffner SD, Wang JC. The pathophysiology and nonsurgical treatment of lumbar spinal stenosis. Instr Course Lect 2009;58:657–68.
16. North American Spine Society. Clinical guidelines for multidisciplinary spine care: diagnosis and treatment of degenerative lumbar spinal stenosis. Burr Ridge (IL): North American Spine Society; 2007.
17. Deyo RA. Drug therapy for back pain: which drugs help patients? Spine 1996;21:2840–9.
18. Cuckler JM, Bernini PA, Wiesel SW, et al. The use of epidural steroids in the treatment of lumbar radicular pain: a prospective, randomized, double-blind study. J Bone Joint Surg Am 1985;67:63–6.
19. Hoogmartens M, Morelle P. Epidural injection in the treatment of spinal stenosis. Acta Orthop Belg 1987;53:409–11.
20. Riew KD, Yin Y, Gilula L, et al. The effect of nerve-root injections on the need for operative treatment of lumbar radicular pain: a prospective, randomized, controlled, double-blind study. J Bone Joint Surg Am 2000;82:1589–93.
21. Riew KD, Park JB, Cho YS, et al. Nerve root blocks in the treatment of lumbar radicular pain: a minimum five-year follow-up. J Bone Joint Surg Am 2006;88: 1722–5.
22. Zucherman JF, Hsu KY, Hartjen CA, et al. A multicenter, prospective, randomized trial evaluating the X STOP interspinous process decompression system for the treatment of neurogenic intermittent claudication: two-year follow-up results. Spine 2005;30:1351–8.
23. Verbiest H. A radicular syndrome from developmental narrowing of the lumbar vertebral canal. J Bone Joint Surg Br 1954;36:230–7.
24. Verbiest H. Results of surgical treatment of idiopathic developmental stenosis of the lumbar vertebral canal. A review of twenty-seven years experience. J Bone Joint Surg Br 1977;59:181–8.
25. Wiltse L, Kirkaldy-Willis W, Ivor GW. The treatment of spinal stenosis. Clin Orthop Relat Res 1976;115: 83–91.

26. Tile M, McNeil SR, Zarins RK, et al. Spinal stenosis: results of treatment. Clin Orthop Relat Res 1976;115: 104–8.

27. Paine KWE. Results of decompression for lumbar spinal stenosis. Clin Orthop 1976;115:96–100.

28. Fast A, Robin CC, Floman Y. Surgical treatment of lumbar spinal stenosis in the elderly. Arch Phys Med Rehabil 1985;66:149–51.

29. Getty CJM. Lumbar spinal stenosis. The clinical spectrum and the results of operation. J Bone Joint Surg Br 1980;62:481–5.

30. Hall S, Bartleson JD, Onofrio B, et al. Lumbar spinal stenosis. Clinical features, diagnostic procedures and results of surgical treatment in 68 patients. Ann Intern Med 1985;103:271–5.

31. Nasca RJ. Surgical management of lumbar spinal stenosis. Spine 1987;12:809–16.

32. Johnsson KE, Rosén I, Udén A. The natural course of lumbar spinal stenosis. Clin Orthop Relat Res 1992;279:82–6.

33. Johnsson KE, Udén A, Rosén I. The effect of decompression on the natural course of spinal stenosis. A comparison of surgically treated and untreated patients. Spine 1991;16:615–9.

34. Katz JN, Lipson SJ, Larson MG, et al. The outcome of decompressive laminectomy for degenerative lumbar stenosis. J Bone Joint Surg Am 1991;73: 809–16.

35. Katz JN, Lipson SJ, Chang LC. Seven to 10-year outcome of decompressive surgery for degenerative lumbar spinal stenosis. Spine 1996;21:92–8.

36. Herno A, Airaksinen O, Saari T, et al. Long-term results of surgical treatment of lumbar spinal stenosis. Spine 1993;18:1471–4.

37. Airaksinen O, Herno A, Turunen V. Surgical outcome of 438 patients treated surgically for lumbar spinal stenosis. Spine 1997;22:2278–82.

38. Cornefjord M, Byröd G, Brisby H, et al. A long-term (4-12 year) follow-up study of surgical treatment of lumbar spinal stenosis. Eur Spine J 2000;9:563–70.

39. Jönsson B, Annertz M, Sjöberg C, et al. A prospective and consecutive study of surgically treated lumbar spinal stenosis. Spine 1997;22:2938–44.

40. Atlas SJ, Deyo RA, Keller RB, et al. The Maine lumbar spine study, part III: 1-year outcomes of surgical and nonsurgical management of lumbar spinal stenosis. Spine 1996;21:1787–95.

41. Atlas SJ, Keller RB, Robson D, et al. Surgical and nonsurgical management of lumbar spinal stenosis. Four year outcomes from the Maine Lumbar Spine Study. Spine 2000;25:556–62.

42. Atlas SJ, Keller RB, Wu YA, et al. Long-term outcomes of surgical and nonsurgical management of lumbar spinal stenosis: 8 to 10 year results from the Maine Lumbar Spine Study. Spine 2005;30:936–43.

43. Amundsen T, Weber H, Nordal HJ, et al. Lumbar spinal stenosis: conservative or surgical management? A prospective 10-year study. Spine 2000;25:1424–35.

44. Mariconda M, Fava R, Gatto A. Unilateral laminectomy for bilateral decompression of lumbar spinal stenosis: a prospective comparative study with conservatively treated patients. J Spinal Disord 2002;15:39–46.

45. Athiviraham A, Yen D. Is spinal stenosis better treated surgically or nonsurgically? Clin Orthop Relat Res 2007;458:90–3.

46. Malmivaara A, Slatis P, Heliovaara M, et al. Surgical or nonoperative treatment for lumbar spinal stenosis. Spine 2007;32:1–8.

47. Weinstein JN, Tosteson TD, Lurie JD, et al. Surgical versus nonsurgical therapy for lumbar spinal stenosis. N Engl J Med 2008;358:794–810.

48. Birkmeyer NJ, Weinstein JN, Tosteson ANA, et al. Design of the Spine Patient Outcomes Research Trial (SPORT). Spine 2002;27:1361–72.

Cervical Spondylotic Myelopathy: A Review of the Evidence

Eric Klineberg, MD

KEYWORDS
- Cervical spondylotic myelopathy
- Corpectomy • Laminectomy • Cervical arthroplasty

Cervical spondylotic myelopathy (CSM) is the most common progressive spinal cord disorder in patients more than 55 years old. More than 50% of middle-aged patients show radiographic evidence of cervical disease, but only 10% have clinically significant root or cord compression. CSM is also the most common cause of acquired spasticity in later life and may lead to progressive spasticity and neurologic decline.[1] There are multiple symptoms of myelopathy, including motor and sensory disturbances, but the onset is usually insidious. Lower extremities are affected first, and patients can complain of gait disturbance, with degeneration of the spinocerebellar and corticospinal tracts. The upper extremities can then become affected with loss of coordination and difficulty with fine motor tasks.[2] However, the symptoms can be much more subtle and may involve axial neck pain, scapular pain, or a progressive broad-based gait. Often, the patient's spouse notices the disturbance earliest as an unfamiliar walking pattern.

GOALS

This article explores some of the controversies in CSM and reviews pertinent articles, specifically prospective and randomized clinical trials when possible, to obtain the cleanest and least biased data. The 4 current controversial topics that surround CSM are: (1) natural history of mild CSM; (2) surgical approach: anterior versus posterior; (3) laminoplasty or laminectomy; and (4) cervical arthroplasty for CSM.

NATURAL HISTORY

The natural history of CSM is not well known. Historically surgical treatment has been the mainstay for progressive CSM. Traction and soft collars have not been shown to alter the natural course of the disease.[3] There have been several series studying patients treated conservatively, and 26% to 50% of patients may deteriorate neurologically over time.[4–7] Clark and Robinson[4] found that 5% of patients deteriorate quickly, 20% have a gradual but steady decline in function, and 70% have a stepwise progression in their symptoms with variable periods of quiescent disease.[4] These patients are also at increased risk of sustaining severe neurologic injuries with even minor trauma.[8] Minor trauma can result in a central cord syndrome or in quadriplegia without fracture or dislocation. Early treatment has also been shown to alter the prognosis in patients.[9–11] treated within 1 year of onset of symptoms.

In 1992, Rowland[12] wrote an editorial for *Neurology* entitled Surgical treatment of CSM: time for a controlled trial. In the article, he pleaded for a randomized controlled trial to study the outcome of these patients. He noted that often patients can be successfully treated nonoperatively and the only way to determine the appropriate surgical intervention and timing, was to conduct a controlled trial. The Cochrane review searched the literature in 2002 and found only 1 randomized controlled trial from 2000 with a 2-year follow-up that specifically addressed the conservative versus operative management of mild CSM.[13,14] They were unable to draw any conclusions based on that study (**Table 1**).

Adult and Pediatric Spinal Surgery, Department of Orthopaedics, 4860 Y Street, Suite 3800, Sacramento, CA 95817, USA
E-mail address: eric.klineberg@ucdmc.ucdavis.edu

Orthop Clin N Am 41 (2010) 193–202
doi:10.1016/j.ocl.2009.12.010

Table 1
Conservative treatment of cervical spondylotic myelopathy

Study	Level of Evidence	Type of Study	Number of Patients	Inclusion Criteria	f/u Time	Outcomes	Conclusions
Kadanka et al,[38] 2000	II	Prospective randomized (coin toss)	48 (21 surgical, 27 conservative)	mJOA ≥ 12, age < 75 y, MRI evidence of compression, no previous surgery	2 y	No change in mJOA, no change in walking	No difference
Kadanka et al,[15] 2002	II	Prospective randomized (coin toss)	68 (35 conservative, 33 surgical-ACDF 22, corpectomy 6, laminoplasty 5)	mJOA ≥ 12, younger than 75 y, MRI evidence of compression, no previous surgery	3 y	No change in mJOA, no change in walking	No advantage
Sampath et al,[16] 2000	III	Prospective questionnaire	62 (31 surgery) f/u for 43/62 (70%)	> 8 wk CSM symptoms, radiographic evidence, age > 18 y	11.2 mo (8–13)	Surgery with improved functional status, neurologic status, = greater satisfaction	Surgery improved outcomes
Matsumoto et al,[17] 2000	III	Retrospective	52	CSM, MRI evidence of compression	3 y (1–6)	No change in JOA, 70% satisfactory results	No difference
Nakamura et al,[18] 1998	IV	Retrospective	64	CSM, > 1 year f/u	f/u 3–10 y	No disability in 30%	Conservative management is OK

Abbreviations: ACDF, anterior cervical discectomy and fusion; f/u, follow-up; mJOA, modified Japanese Orthopedic Association; MRI, magnetic resonance imaging.

That study was expanded and now has 3-year follow-up data.[15] Those 2 studies are the only randomized controlled studies that attempt to determine the role of surgical intervention for mild CSM. The 3-year study by Kadanka and colleagues[15] followed 68 patients prospectively in a randomized controlled trial, and no patients were lost to follow-up. Randomization was accomplished by a coin toss and patients were randomized to surgical decompression or conservative management. Conservative management consisted of a soft collar, nonsteroidal antiinflammatory drugs (NSAIDS), and discouragement from high-risk activities. Surgical management was at the surgeon's discretion. The inclusion criteria were mild myelopathy, that is, modified Japanese Orthopedic Association (mJOA) score greater than 12, younger than 75 years, and evidence of cervical compression on magnetic resonance imaging (MRI). The disease in these patients was mild; the median cord compression was 71 mm², and most had only 1 level disease for a median duration of 1 year in the nonsurgical group and a median of 3 years in the surgical group. The procedure used for decompression in 67% (22/33) of the patients was a 1-level anterior discectomy and fusion. The outcome measures included mJOA, timed 10-m walk, and evaluation of daily activities that were collected preintervention and at regular postoperative intervals until final follow-up. There were no statistically significant changes in mJOA or walking scores from pre- and postintervention and no significant changes between the operative and nonoperative groups. There was a slight but significant difference in deterioration of the conservatively treated group in their activities of daily living. The investigators' conclusions were that for mild CSM nonoperative treatment was as effective as surgical decompression, and that patients can be successfully treated nonoperatively for up to 3 years. Although there are some problems with the study (randomization by coin toss), it is a compelling argument for nonoperative management for mild CSM.

A prospective questionnaire was used by Sampath and colleagues[16] for mild CSM treated surgically and nonsurgically. Sixty-two patients were enrolled, however only 43 (69%) completed the study at an average of 11.2 months follow-up (8–13 months). The investigators noted that surgery was associated with improved functional status and improved neurologic status, which correlated directly with patient satisfaction.

Two retrospective studies focused on the long-term outcome of patients with CSM treated non-operatively. Matsumoto and colleagues[17] reported on 52 patients with an average 3-year follow-up (1–6 years). These patients had 70% satisfaction and no significant deterioration in their JOA scores. Nakamura and colleagues[18] reported on 64 patients with a follow-up of 3–10 years with 30% of patients reporting no disability. The conclusion made by both investigators was that mild CSM could be treated successfully with conservative measures for a significant number of patients. They noted that deterioration may occur over time and these patients need to be followed closely for signs of neurologic injury.

Most investigators suggest that there are multiple factors that play a role in the success of operative or nonoperative management of CSM. Several papers have provided multivariate analysis on the successful operative and nonoperative patients.[19,20] Their conclusions are similar. Patients may be successfully treated conservatively if they have lower mJOA scores, minimal neurologic findings (normal central motor conduction times), spinal transverse area greater than 70 mm², and are older patients. Surgery was successful for patients with more severe neurologic symptoms, a hyperintense signal on MRI with localized disease and who had canal expansion greater than 40% postoperatively, and were of younger age.

The author's approach to these patients follows the literature closely. I place a great deal of emphasis on the clinical examination and on the patient's function. If the disease is mild and the symptoms are mild, I prefer to watch these patients closely with regular scheduled visits. If the patient has significant symptoms of myelopathy, including walking and balance difficulty, poor hand coordination, or progressive neurologic decline, I favor early surgical decompression.

SURGICAL APPROACH

There are multiple surgical approaches to treat cervical myelopathy. The principle goal of any approach is to increase the canal diameter and provide the cord with adequate room to avoid static or dynamic compression. This can improve or prevent the decline of neurologic function if done early enough in the disease. However, there are multiple factors that must be taken into account when considering anterior versus posterior decompression.[21]

Cervical sagittal alignment is an important consideration because it affects the type of surgical approach. In kyphotic spines, posterior decompression will not allow the spinal cord to drift posteriorly and may increase the tension on the spinal cord if the kyphosis progresses.[22] It is not always possible to correct the sagittal alignment through a posterior approach; anterior

Table 2
Anterior versus posterior approach

Study	Level of Evidence	Type of Study	Number of Patients	Inclusion Criteria	f/u Time	Outcomes	Conclusions
Kristof et al,[38] 2009	III	Retrospective	103 patients(42 anterior fusion, 61 posterior fusion)	Greater than 2-level CSM disease	Anterior (16 y, posterior 5.4 y)	No significant difference in: surgical complications, medical complications, mortality, change in Nurick score, change in neck pain, change in cobb angle, patient satisfaction	no difference between approaches
Iwasaki et al,[26] 2007	III	Retrospective	22 Anterior corpectomy, 66 laminoplasty	OPLL	Anterior 6 y, laminoplasty 10 y	Anterior: improved neurologic outcomes (JOA and recovery rate) with OPLL > 60% occupying lesion or hill-shaped lesion. More complications in anterior: 15% graft, 26% required. surgery	Anterior surgery with improved results for severe OPLL and compression
Edwards et al,[23] 2002	III	Retrospective matched cohort	64 multilevel corpectomy, 26 laminoplasty.	> 3 levels, no prior surgery, no instability, experienced surgeons (13 from each group were matched)	Anterior 49 mo, posterior 40 mo	No significant difference in: change in Nurick scores, subjective improvement, neck pain, 38% adjacent level disease with corpectomy, 8% with laminoplasty. Complications: anterior 9/13, 4 with dysphagia, laminoplasty 1 C5 palsy, 1 wound dehiscence	Laminoplasty safer

Wada et al,[25] 2001	Retrospective	III	CSM, JOA < 13, compression on imaging	23 subtotal corpectomy and 24 laminoplasty, no significant difference for preoperative risk factors (JOA, age, spinal cord compression)	Corpectomy 15 y, laminoplasty 11.7 y	No significant difference between groups. Improved JOA scores maintained at > 10y Complications: anterior 54% adjacent disease, 26% with pseudo, laminoplasty 3 with kyphosis, axial neck pain in 40%	Both with complications, both effective up to 10 y
Yonenobu et al,[24] 1992	Retrospective	III	Multilevel CSM	48 (41 with f/u) subtotal corpectomy, 52 (42 with f/u) laminoplasty	Anterior 53 mo, post 43 mo	No significance in any outcome measure: JOA, rate of recovery. More complications in anterior (12 vs 3) including. 10 graft complications	Laminoplasty is safer with no change in outcome

Abbreviations: f/u, follow-up; OPLL, ossified posterior longitudinal ligament.

reconstruction with lordotic spacers may allow the patient to regain cervical lordosis. Fusion of the spine in a kyphotic position increases the abnormal forces on the vertebral column and may lead to increased degeneration and further disk disease. There is no clear evidence that either anterior or posterior decompression more reliably affects recovery from myelopathy. However, the location of compression does dictate the most direct approach to cord decompression.

Anterior Versus Posterior

Several studies have assessed the advantage or disadvantage of anterior and posterior cervical approaches to treat CSM. None are randomized and none are prospective (**Table 2**).

Edwards and colleagues[23] published a retrospective report on a matched cohort of anterior corpectomy versus laminoplasty. Sixty-four patients met the inclusion criteria that included functional loss consistent with CSM, greater than 3 levels of disease, no prior surgery, no evidence of instability, and surgery that was performed by experienced surgeons. Thirteen from each group were then matched for age, preoperative Nurick grade, and sagittal alignment. Follow-up for these patients was for an average of 40 months. At the latest follow-up, there were no significant difference in change in Nurick grades, with both groups showing lasting improvement by 1 grade. Similarly, there was improvement in each group for subjective neural outcome and neck pain that was not statistically significant. There was no difference in the ability to decompress the canal, and although the motion was decreased for both groups, it tended to be greater for the corpectomy group (57%) than for the laminoplasty group (38%). There was, however, a significant difference in complications. The anterior corpectomy group had 9/13 patients with complications including 4 who had dysphagia that persisted after 2 years. The laminoplasty group that had 1 late disk herniation that required *anterior cervical discectomy and fusion* (ACDF) 6 months after the laminoplasty. However, in the laminoplasty group as a whole (ie, prematching), there was 1 transient C5 root palsy and 1 wound dehiscence. In addition, the anterior group had a 38% risk of adjacent level disease compared with 8% in the laminoplasty group. This may relate to the maintenance of motion in the cervical spine, however, this is not yet known. The conclusions made by the investigators stated that the anterior and posterior approaches have similar clinical outcomes, with a significant increase in early and late complications from the anterior approach.

This finding was similar to several other retrospective reviews. In 1992, Yonenobu and colleagues[24] published a report on 100 patients followed for an average of 4 years with no change in outcome measures. There was again significant morbidity associated with the anterior approach. The Yonenobu group published an extended follow-up with 15 years for the corpectomy group and an average of 11.7 years for the laminoplasty group and reported improved JOA outcome scores that persisted.[25] They noted 54% adjacent level disease and a 26% pseudarthrosis rate in the corpectomy group. One of the 24 patients in the laminoplasty group (4%) went on to develop kyphosis without clinical symptoms. However, 40% of the laminoplasty patients complained of neck pain compared with 15% of the corpectomy group. The investigators' conclusions were that both procedures provided long-term benefit, and that both groups had major disadvantages.

The same group of investigators analyzed the effects of an ossified posterior longitudinal ligament (OPLL) and stratified the patients based on the amount of neural compression.[26] They separated the corpectomy and laminoplasty groups on the basis of anterior compression that occupied greater than 60% of the canal, and also characterized the morphology of the compression. They noted that the anterior decompression group with an occupying lesion greater than 60% improved from a mean JOA of 9.3 to 13.4, compared with the laminoplasty group, which improved from 9.4 to 11.0; this difference was significant. They also noted worse outcomes for patients who underwent laminoplasty for hill-shaped lesions compared with plateau-shaped lesions. There was no difference for these lesions in the anterior group. There were more complications in the corpectomy group, including 15% graft complications and a 26% rate of additional surgery. Despite the greater complications, the investigators recommended anterior decompression for hill-shaped lesions with more than 60% canal compromise.

These studies suggest that anterior corpectomy may be preferred for patients with severe anterior disease (OPLL > 60%) and severe compression. Similar outcomes are seen with patients with more limited disease compared with laminoplasty. Anterior surgery has significant complications including dysphagia, nonunion, and adjacent level disease. Laminoplasty avoids the risks associated with the anterior approach and the risks associated with fusion, but may lead to continued cervical pain. Several articles assess the advantages of types of posterior surgical approach.

LAMINOPLASTY, LAMINECTOMY, AND LAMINECTOMY AND FUSION

Three retrospective papers have examined the preferred method of posterior decompression: laminectomy, laminectomy and fusion, or laminoplasty (**Table 3**). The data from these papers are similar. The posterior approach was found to appropriately decompress the spinal canal regardless of method. However, laminoplasty was found to be safer with less early and late complications than laminectomy alone or laminectomy and fusion. Patient satisfaction for laminectomy (66% good or excellent) was inferior to that for laminoplasty (86%) or anterior surgery (92%), despite a 37% nonunion rate for the anterior surgery.[27] Complications in the laminectomy group were progressive postoperative kyphosis, which occurred in 5/22 (23%) patients.[28] Complications in the laminectomy and fusion group were related to fusion and this group had the same rate of postoperative neck pain as the laminoplasty group (69%).[29]

My decisions regarding approach are related to the location and extent of disease, the overall alignment of the cervical spine, and amount of cervical pain. Discrete ventral disease with anterior osteophytes and disk herniations should be approached ventrally for adequate decompression and preservation of the neural elements. Dorsal compression with ligamentum flavum hypertrophy should be approached dorsally. This allows for direct decompression. Often CSM is diffuse without an obvious single level of disease, and for these cases a dorsal approach can better decompress multiple levels.

The extent of the disease also plays a role in determining the approach used. For discrete 1 or 2 level disease, most surgeons, like the author, prefer an anterior approach.[30,31] If there is significant OPLL (ie, >60%) then a corpectomy may be used to allow safe decompression of the neural elements. For multilevel disease, a posterior approach allows excellent visualization of the neural elements and an extensile decompression.

Cervical kyphosis may occur with posterior surgery, even with preservation of the posterior elements as in laminoplasty. If the cervical spine is neutral to lordosis then the laminoplasty procedure for multilevel disease is preferred. If there is focal kyphosis, then an ACDF for focal correction followed by laminoplasty may also be considered. Significant kyphosis usually requires an anterior

Table 3
Laminectomy and laminoplasty

Study	Level of Evidence	Type of Study	Number of Patients	Inclusion	f/u Time	Outcomes	Conclusions
Heller et al,[29] 2001	III	Retrospective matched cohort	32 LE+F 26 LP 50 met inclusion	CSM, cord compression, no instability, experienced surgeon: 13 matched for age, duration, Nurick	LE+F 25.5 mo, LP 26.2 mo	Improved Nurick scores, subjective neck pain 9/13 in both groups, loss of motion: LE+F 69% LP 35% LE+F: 14 complications in 9 patients, progression of myelopathy in 2	Laminoplasty better and safer than laminectomy and fusion
Kaminsky et al,[28] 2004	III	Retrospective	20 LP 22 LE	> 2 levels of CSM, myelopathic	LP 65.4 mo, LE 64.8	No difference in pain, neck stiffness Nurick better in laminoplasty, but scores started higher (P>.0001). Complications: LP: 2 C5 palsy, LE 5 with kyphosis	Laminoplasty better or as good as laminectomy, fewer complication
Herkowitz et al,[27] 1988	III	Retrospective	45 patients 18 anterior, 12 LE 15 LP	3 level disease, 2-y f/u	2-year f/u	Anterior 92% excellent or good, LE 66% excellent or good, LP 86% excellent or good, loss of lordosis in LE group. Complications: 37% nonunion in anterior, LE 3 pts with kyphosis 2 required. Anterior fusion, 2 patients with hinge closure in LP required. revision surgery	Laminectomy inferior to anterior approach or laminoplasty

Abbreviations: f/u, follow-up; LP, laminoplasty; LE, laminectomy; LE+F, laminectomy + fusion.

and posterior fusion for adequate decompression and stabilization.

For patients with significant neck pain the anterior approach is favored.. Progressive CSM is a disease of cervical compression and neurologic decline, and the associated cervical pain is of secondary importance. Therefore, laminoplasty with its ability to address multiple levels, and limited short- and long-term morbidity, despite neck pain, is the author's procedure of choice.

CERVICAL ARTHROPLASTY

Motion preservation is an old idea that is gaining new popularity. Decompression procedures that allow more space for the cord while either limiting the fusion or maintaining segmental motion by placing disk arthroplasty devices have been hypothesized to decrease the incidence of adjacent level disease. Several studies have looked at this issue of adjacent segment disease and Hilibrand and colleagues[32] reported the incidence of 3% per year. Whether adjacent level degeneration is the result of the fusion, or simply the expression of the natural deterioration of the motion segments, is unknown. Biomechanical studies have shown increased intradiscal pressures above and below the fusion, but this has yet to be correlated clinically.[33]

In 2008, Riew and colleagues[34] combined the data from 2 prospective randomized trials that compared ACDF versus cervical arthroplasty (**Table 4**). They combined the data from the US Food and Drug Administration Investigational Device Exemption studies on Prestige ST and Bryan artificial disk replacements (both manufactured by Medtronic Inc, Memphis, TN, USA). Eighty-eight patients from the Bryan study and 111 patients from the Prestige ST trial met the inclusion criteria of myelopathy and spondylosis from retrodiscal pathology at a single level, Nurick score greater than 1, no instability, and no segmental kyphosis. Of these 199 patients 106 underwent disk arthroplasty and 93 underwent ACDF at 1 level. Postoperative follow-up was undertaken for 2 years, and no patients were lost to follow-up. Both groups had Neck Disability Index (NDI) improvement of greater than 15 points, and Short Form-36 (SF-36) scores that improved greater than 15 points. In the Prestige ST group 89% of the arthroplasty patients and 81% of the arthrodesis patients had improvement or maintenance of neurologic function for the 2 years; similar findings were reported for the Bryan group. None of these findings were significant between the 2 groups at 2 years. The investigators concluded that for limited disease, disk arthroplasty performed as well as a single-level fusion for neurologic function,

Table 4
Cervical arthroplasty

Study	Level of Evidence	Type of Study	Number of Patients	Inclusion	f/u Time	Outcomes	Conclusions
Riew et al,[34] 2008	I	Prospective randomized	199: 106 TDR-Bryan and Prestige ST, 93 arthrodesis	Single-level CSM, Nurick > 1, no instability, no kyphosis	24 months	NDI improved >15, SF-36 improved > 15, no statistically difference between groups	TDR same as fusion for one-level compression
Sekhon,[36] 2004	IV	Case series	11 patients with 15 Bryan TDR	One-or two-level CSM	5 patients followed for 18 mo	NDI improve 45%, improve 1 Nurick grade. Complications: 1 fusion at 17 mo, 1 focal kyphosis with worsening of symptoms	TDR can be successfully used for limited CSM

Abbreviations: f/u, follow-up; NDI, Neck Disability Index; SF-36, Short Form-36; TDR, total disk replacement.

satisfaction, and neck pain. No conclusions were reached regarding adjacent level degeneration in this short-term follow-up study.

Sekhon[35–37] has also published several case series where he followed 11 patients with 15 Bryan artificial disk replacements. However, only 5 were followed for 18 months.[36] He found that the patients' NDI improved 45%, and by 1 Nurick grade. He had 1 spontaneous fusion at 17 months and 1 patient who developed focal kyphosis and transient worsening of their symptoms. He concluded that cervical arthroplasty may be a reasonable alternative to fusion for limited CSM.

The author has treated limited anterior pathology CSM with a single-level ACDF. Although the data regarding outcome at 2 years are encouraging, longer follow-up is needed to justify the added expense of arthroplasty and the potential for future complications, including wear debris and recurrent stenosis at the same level. ACDF is also practical. Despite excellent randomized controlled trials demonstrating equivalency, few insurance providers provide authorization and patients are unable or unwilling to bear the cost themselves.

SUMMARY

Randomized clinical studies provide the greatest information with the least amount of bias. These studies allow the effect of treatment to be determined and the most appropriate solution to be chosen. CSM is a complex disease with many operative and nonoperative solutions. Controversy exists regarding timing of treatment, approach, technique, and modern devices. However, despite these controversies, few randomized controlled studies exist. This high level of research is needed.

REFERENCES

1. Rao R. Neck pain, cervical radiculopathy and cervical myelopathy. J Bone Joint Surg Am 2002; 84(10):1872–81.
2. Geck MJ, Eismont FJ. Surgical options for the treatment of cervical spondylotic myelopathy. Orthop Clin North Am 2002;33(2):329–48.
3. McCormick WE, Steinmetz MP, Benzel EC. Cervical spondylotic myelopathy: make the difficult diagnosis then refer for surgery. Cleve Clin J Med 2003;70(10): 899–904.
4. Clarke E, Robinson PK. Cervical myelopathy: a complication of cervical spondylosis. Brain 1956; 79(3):483–510.
5. Epstein JA. The surgical management of cervical spinal stenosis, spondylosis, and myeloradiculopathy by means of the posterior approach. Spine 1988; 13(7):864–9.
6. Syman L, Lavender P. The surgical treatment of cervical spondylotic myelopathy. Neurology 1967; 17:117–26.
7. Roberts AH. Myelopathy due to cervical spondylosis treated by collar immobilization. Neurology 1966;16: 951–4.
8. Epstein N, Epstein JA, Benjamin V, et al. Traumatic myelopathy in patients with cervical spinal stenosis without fracture or dislocation. Spine 1980;5:489–96.
9. Montgomery DM, Brower RS. Cervical spondylotic myelopathy. Clinical syndrome and natural history. Orthop Clin North Am 1992;23(3):487–93.
10. Phillips DG. Surgical treatment of myelopathy with cervical spondylosis. J Neurol Neurosurg Psychiatr 1973;36(5):879–84.
11. Ebersold MJ, Pare MC, Quast LM. Surgical treatment for cervical spondylotic myelopathy. J Neurosurg 1995;82(5):745–51.
12. Rowland LP. Surgical treatment of cervical spondylotic myelopathy: time for a controlled trial. Neurology 1992;42(1):5–13.
13. Fouyas IP, Statham PF, Sandercock PA. Cochrane review on the role of surgery in cervical spondylotic radiculomyelopathy. Spine (Phila Pa 1976) 2002; 27(7):736–47.
14. Kadanka Z, Bednarík J, Vohánka S, et al. Conservative treatment versus surgery in spondylotic cervical myelopathy: a prospective randomised study. Eur Spine J 2000;9(6):538–44.
15. Kadanka Z, Mares M, Bednaník J, et al. Approaches to spondylotic cervical myelopathy: conservative versus surgical results in a 3-year follow-up study. Spine 2002;27(20):2205–10.
16. Sampath P, Bendebba M, Davis JD, et al. Outcome of patients treated for cervical myelopathy: a prospective, multicenter study with independent clinical review. Spine 2000;25:670–6.
17. Matsumoto M, Toyama Y, Ishikawa M, et al. Increased signal intensity of the spinal cord on magnetic resonance images in cervical compressive myelopathy: does it predict the outcome of conservative treatment? Spine 2000;25:677–82.
18. Nakamura K, Kurokawa T, Hoshino Y, et al. Conservative treatment for cervical spondylotic myelopathy: achievement and sustainability of a level of "no disability". J Spinal Disord 1998;11(2):175–9.
19. Uchida K, Nakajima H, Sato R, et al. Multivariate analysis of the neurological outcome of surgery for cervical compressive myelopathy. J Orthop Sci 2005;10(6):564–73.
20. Kadanka Z, Mares M, Bednarík J, et al. Predictive factors for mild forms of spondylotic cervical myelopathy treated conservatively or surgically. Eur J Neurol 2005;12(1):16–24.

21. Edwards CC II, Riew D, Anderson PA, et al. Cervical myelopathy: current diagnostic and treatment strategies. Spine J 2003;3:68–81.

22. Sodeyama T, Goto S, Mochizuki M, et al. Effect of decompression enlargement laminoplasty for posterior shifting of the spinal cord. Spine 1999;24(15): 1527–31.

23. Edwards CC 2nd, Heller JG, Murakami H. Corpectomy versus laminoplasty for multilevel cervical myelopathy: an independent matched-cohort analysis. Spine (Phila Pa 1976) 2002;27(11):1168–75.

24. Yonenobu K, Hosono N, Iwasaki M, et al. Laminoplasty versus subtotal corpectomy. A comparative study of results in multisegmental cervical spondylotic myelopathy. Spine 1992;17(11):1281–4.

25. Wada E, Suzuki S, Kanazawa A, et al. Subtotal corpectomy versus laminoplasty for multilevel cervical spondylotic myelopathy: a long-term follow-up study over 10 years. Spine (Phila Pa 1976) 2001;26(13):1443–7.

26. Iwasaki M, Okuda S, Miyauchi A, et al. Surgical strategy for cervical myelopathy due to ossification of the posterior longitudinal ligament: Part 2: Advantages of anterior decompression and fusion over laminoplasty. Spine 2007;32(6):654–60.

27. Herkowitz HN. A comparison of anterior cervical fusion, cervical laminectomy, and cervical laminoplasty for the surgical management of multiple level spondylotic radiculopathy. Spine 1988;13(7):774–80.

28. Kaminsky SB, Clark CR, Traynelis VC. Operative treatment of cervical spondylotic myelopathy and radiculopathy. A comparison of laminectomy and laminoplasty at five year average follow-up. Iowa Orthop J 2004;24:95–105.

29. Heller JG, Edwards CC 2nd, Murakami H, et al. Laminoplasty versus laminectomy and fusion for multilevel cervical myelopathy: an independent matched cohort analysis. Spine 2001;26(12): 1330–6.

30. Yonenobu K, Fuji T, Ono K, et al. Choice of surgical treatment for multisegmental cervical spondylotic myelopathy. Spine 1985;10(8):710–6.

31. Herkowitz HN, Kurz LT, Overholt DP. Surgical management of cervical soft disc herniation. A comparison between the anterior and posterior approach. Spine 1990;15(10):1026–30.

32. Hilibrand AS, Carlson GD, Palumbo MA, et al. Radiculopathy and myelopathy at segments adjacent to the site of a previous anterior cervical arthrodesis. J Bone Joint Surg Am 1999;81(4):519–28.

33. Eck JC, Humphreys SC, Lim TH, et al. Biomechanical study on the effect of cervical spine fusion on adjacent-level intradiscal pressure and segmental motion. Spine 2002;27(22):2431–4.

34. Riew KD, Buchowski JM, Sasso R, et al. Cervical disc arthroplasty compared with arthrodesis for the treatment of myelopathy. J Bone Joint Surg Am 2008;90(11):2354–64.

35. Sekhon LH. Cervical arthroplasty in the management of spondylotic myelopathy. J Spinal Disord Tech 2003;16:307–13.

36. Sekhon LH. Cervical arthroplasty in the management of spondylotic myelopathy: 18-month results. Neurosurg Focus 2004;17:E8.

37. Sekhon LH. Two-level artificial disc placement for spondylotic cervical myelopathy. J Clin Neurosci 2004;11:412–5.

38. Kristof RA, Kiefer T, Thudium M, et al. Comparison of ventral corpectomy and plate-screw-instrumented fusion with dorsal laminectomy and rod-screw-instrumented fusion for treatment of at least two vertebral-level spondylotic cervical myelopathy. Eur Spine J 2009;18(12):1951–6.

Dynamic Constructs for Spinal Fusion: An Evidence-Based Review

Michael P. Kelly, MD[a],*, James M. Mok, MD[b],
Sigurd Berven, MD[a]

KEYWORDS

- Spinal • Fusion • Dynamic • Rigid • Flexible

Arthrodesis of the spine is an important and useful technique for the management of spinal disorders including deformity, trauma, segmental instability, and symptomatic disc degeneration.[1] Rigid stabilization of the spine with segmental fixation, fixed axis screws, and large diameter rods creates a mechanical environment that is associated with higher fusion rates than noninstrumented or semi-rigid constructs.[2–4] However, rigid segmental fixation may have significant adverse effects including an increase in the stress on adjacent mobile segments, and stress shielding the bone graft material within the regenerate.[5–8] Dynamic stabilization of a painful motion segment is an alternative to rigid internal fixation that may be useful in improving rates of fusion, or in providing an alternative approach to the surgical management of a painful motion segment without arthrodesis. Techniques of dynamic stabilization have been developed and evaluated for the treatment of degenerative conditions of the cervical and lumbar spine, and for thoracolumbar trauma and deformity. The purpose of this article is to review and assess the evidence in the literature on the efficacy of dynamic stabilization techniques in the management of spinal disorders.

Dynamic stabilization of the spine is a mechanical constraint of spinal motion that allows selective motion of the functional spinal unit. Dynamic stabilization in the cervical spine with a dynamic plating system is intended to limit motion to compression without translation. Selective compression may improve interbody healing and fusion mass formation.[9] In the lumbar spine, posterior dynamic stabilization devices may provide segmental distraction without fusion, or may limit the motion of an unstable motion segment. When not used for fusion, these devices are designed to be load sharing with the spinal segment, selectively reducing translatory stresses and potentially modifying axial pain. Dynamic stabilization encompasses motion-sparing options for spinal instrumentation. Total disc arthroplasty devices have limited constraint in flexion, extension, and rotation compared with the normal motion segment. Rigid fixation of a motion segment causes changes in motion segment kinematics in the adjacent segments and increases in the area of center axis of rotation and intradiscal pressure. Less constrained motion-sparing options, including total disc arthroplasty in the cervical and lumbar spine, may reduce the effect of instrumentation on adjacent segments.[10] The association of adjacent segment degeneration and disease with altered segmental kinematics remains controversial. The efficacy of restoring kinemetics of the adjacent segment with motion-sparing devices on reducing adjacent segment

Disclosures: Sigurd Berven, MD; Consultancies: Medtronic, DePuy, Biomet, Osteotech, Pioneer, US Spine, Research/Institutional Support: Medtronic, DePuy, AO Spine, Royalties: Medtronic, Osteotech.
[a] Department of Orthopaedic Surgery, University of California, 500 Parnassus Avenue, MU 320-W, San Francisco, CA 94110, USA
[b] The Spine Institute, 1301 20th Street, Suite 400, Santa Monica, CA 90404, USA
* Corresponding author.
E-mail address: kellym@orthosurg.ucsf.edu

Orthop Clin N Am 41 (2010) 203–215
doi:10.1016/j.ocl.2009.12.004

degeneration and pathology has yet to be reported in long-term follow-up.[11]

This article is a systematic review of the evidence for dynamic stabilization devices used for cervical fusion and lumbar posterior dynamic stabilization for degenerative disease and trauma. Selection of devices for discussion was limited to dynamic stabilization options with published clinical outcome studies, and including objective patient-based health-related quality of life outcomes. All devices included have been approved by the US Food and Drug Administration (FDA) through 510k regulatory provision. The studies of lumbar and thoracolumbar posterior dynamic stabilization devices include physician-directed, or off-label uses of the devices without fusion. The quality of the evidence is graded using the technique of the Center for Evidence-based Medicine.[11,12] The article is intended to provide the reader with an overview of published evidence of efficacy for dynamic stabilization devices in the cervical and lumbar spine.

CERVICAL SPINE

Anterior cervical plating is associated with decreased rates of graft dislodgement, kyphosis, and endplate fracture, and increased rates of fusion following multilevel anterior cervical discectomy and fusion.[13,14] Rigid plating of multilevel constructs is believed to increase fusion rates by minimizing micromotion at the interbody spaces.[14] With more than 2 treated levels, however, reported pseudarthrosis rates have been similar for instrumented and noninstrumented constructs.[15] The rigid anterior cervical plate may prevent segmental subsidence, and loading of the interbody graft, allowing for gap formation and leading to nonunion. Dynamic cervical fusion plates are designed to compress the graft axially while preventing translation. There are 3 main types marketed and studied that are designed to load the interbody graft with variable axis of screws or axial compression capacity in the plate design.[16] The first allows load sharing through screws that may toggle within the plate, allowing for compression through the graft. A second allows for graft compression through sliding screws within the plate, as the screw holes are oblong (Fig. 1). A third design allows for rigid fixation through the screw holes, and allows for shortening of the plate itself through a telescoping design.

The biomechanical advantages of a dynamic cervical plate have been validated in basic scientific investigations. In a cadaveric C5 corpectomy model, Reidy and colleagues[17] compared compressive forces borne by rigid and dynamic cervical plates. With optimally sized grafts, the rigid plate bore 23% of the load, versus 9% for the dynamic plate. The interbody graft handled 23% more force with the dynamic plate, which supports the intent of loading the interbody graft. With an undersized graft, a situation similar to graft subsidence or contact osteolysis, the dynamic plate allowed for more force transmission through the graft, although the greatest increases in forces were seen in the posterior elements. Brodke and colleagues,[18] in a subsequent C5 corpectomy model, showed a significant increase in the load borne by the rigid plate with graft subsidence. In this model, graft subsidence did not affect the load-sharing properties of a dynamic cervical plate.

Clinical efficacy of dynamic cervical plates has been studied in several retrospective and prospective studies including prospective randomized controlled trials. Epstein[19] reported on 42 patients undergoing single-level anterior cervical disc fusion (ACDF) with a dynamic plate. The results confirmed excellent fusion rates, and documented compression of the graft construct beneath the plate. However, the plate failure rate was 9.5%. Similar results were reported by Casha and Fehlings[20] in their study of dynamic plating for cervical fusion. The cases reviewed were not limited to single-level ACDF, however, and included nearly equal numbers of single- and multilevel ACDF and single- and multilevel corpectomy. They reported an overall fusion rate of 93.8% at 2 years follow-up, with an implant complication rate of 8.2%. Implant failure correlated with an increasing length of construct. Radiographic measurements confirmed the dynamic properties of the plate.

Pitzen and colleagues[21] presented level I data from a trial of 132 patients, comparing rigid with dynamic cervical plating for 1- and 2-level ACDF for degenerative disease or cervical trauma. The outcomes assessed were implant-related complication rates, time to radiographic fusion, loss of lordosis, and outcomes as assessed by the Visual Analog Scale (VAS) and the Neck Disability Index (NDI). The rigid plating group experienced a significantly higher rate of implant complications including plate loosening and screw breakage ($P = .045$) The rigid plating group did have better preservation of cervical lordosis at 2 years follow-up ($P = .003$). There were no significant differences in the clinical outcomes assessments. Because of the difference in complication rates, and despite the differences in cervical lordosis, the investigators concluded that dynamic plates are the preferable method of fixation for 1- and 2-level ACDF.

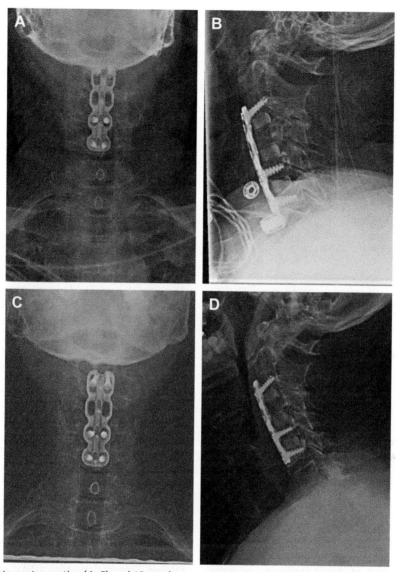

Fig. 1. Immediate postoperative (*A, B*) and 12-week postoperative (*C, D*) anteroposterior and lateral radiographs show settling of the construct, with compression of the interbody grafts. The patient is a 63-year-old woman treated with C3-C6 anterior cervical disc fusion (ACDF) for cervical degenerative disc disease. (*Courtesy of* Phil Weinstein, MD, San Francisco, CA.)

Nunley and colleagues[22] performed a randomized controlled trial of a heterogeneous mix of patients undergoing single- or multilevel ACDF with rigid or dynamic fixation. They found no difference in outcomes for the groups undergoing single-level ACDF, but did find an advantage to dynamic instrumentation for multilevel ACDF. In contrast, DuBois and colleagues[23] reviewed 52 patients undergoing 2- and 3-level ACDF, comparing rigid with dynamic anterior cervical plating. They found an increase in the rate of nonunion when using the dynamic cervical plate ($P = .05$). They measured the amount of construct settling over 1 to 2 years, and found no difference

between the plating systems, thus questioning the compressive properties of the plate in vivo. Clinical outcomes were similar among the groups, which led the investigators to conclude that the more expensive dynamic plates do not offer any clear benefit compared with rigid plates.

Anterior cervical plating is associated with adjacent-level ossification which may be due to impingement from the plate on the adjacent level disc space (**Fig. 2**).[24,25] Although comparative series have shown no difference in incidence of this complication when comparing rigid with dynamic cervical plating, special attention must be paid to technique when using a dynamic

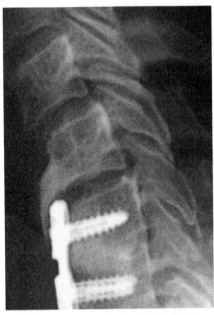

Fig. 2. Adjacent-level ossification due to impingement of the plate at the adjacent disc space. (© 2007 American Academy of Orthopaedic Surgeons. *Reprinted from* the Journal of the American Academy of Orthopaedic Surgeons, volume 15(11), p. 640–6; with permission.)

plate.[16,23] Park and colleagues[26] noted that the incidence of moderate to severe adjacent-level ossification was increased with less than 5 mm of space between the adjacent disc and plate. The implication for those using dynamic plates is that the subsidence of the bodies and graft must be accounted for at the time of surgery, as the plates may encroach on the adjacent levels in follow-up, as the graft is compressed. This problem requires the surgeon to know the amount of subsidence allowed by the plate, and to understand the method of dynamization to optimize plate and screw placement.

Conclusion

The clinical evidence for cervical dynamic plating remains mixed. The literature supports a compressive role of the dynamic cervical plate (**Table 1**). However, there is little evidence for improvement of fusion rates or clinical outcomes compared with rigid fixation. The loss of segmental lordosis and potential for adjacent segment impingement is a significant limitation of cervical dynamic stabilization.

LUMBAR SPINE

The advent of rigid spinal instrumentation was accompanied by higher fusion rates in the treatment of degenerative lumbar disease without clear improvements in clinical outcomes.[29–31] Rigid instrumentation does result in increased forces at the adjacent segments of the spine as measured by intradiscal pressure. The role of increased forces at the adjacent segments in causing adjacent segment degeneration and disease remains undetermined. The rates of adjacent segment disease are as high as 36%.[32] The concern for adjacent segment degeneration and disease has driven the development of dynamic, or semirigid, constructs for lumbar spine instrumentation. As with cervical spine instrumentation, the dynamic instrumentation for the lumbar spine is designed to be a load-sharing device, allowing for fusion without excessive rigidity leading to adjacent segment complications.[33] Some dynamic constructs have also been used without fusion. Preclinical evidence to support less rigid stabilization as a mechanism for improving fusion rates in the spine is limited. In the United States, the FDA has approved lumbar dynamic stabilization devices through the 510k regulatory pathway. A new technology that is substantially equivalent to existing devices that have been in use since before 1976 may be approved by the FDA under the process of 510(k) approval. The US FDA 510(k) regulatory process specifically applies to devices and technologies for which there was a predicate device in existence before 1976. The level of clinical evidence required for 510k approval is variable and approval may be based on mechanical and preclinical studies alone. Dynamic stabilization devices without fusion have been applied in a physician-directed use, or off-label application. Therefore, the literature on lumbar dynamic stabilization without fusion is limited to a few prospective studies. This section reviews the evidence for these devices as instruments for spinal fusion, and discusses the use of fusion devices for dynamic stabilization. For a broader review of the recent data, the reader is referred to the recent publication by Bono and colleagues.[34]

The dynamic systems approved for spinal fusion under the FDA 510k provision are pedicle screw–based constructs that are semirigid, or allow constrained motion in compression or flexion and extension. The rigidity of these constructs is affected by the choice of material and design of the rods connecting pedicle screws. Although solid stainless steel and titanium are commonly used in spinal fusion constructs, the semirigid constructs include polyetheretherketone (PEEK) rods, nitinol rods, specially cut rods (eg, Accuflex), articulated rods, and polyethylene terephthalate cords (Dynesys).[33,35–37] The optimal mechanical

Table 1
Review of clinical evidence for dynamic cervical plating

Authors	Year	Study Design	Indications	Results	Grade of Evidence
Epstein[19]	2003	Retrospective cohort	Degenerative disk disease (DDD), ossification of the posterior longitudinal ligament (OPLL), spondylosis	Mean Nurick score improved 2.5 points; 90.5% fusion rate	C
Casha and Fehlings[20]	2003	Prospective cohort	Spondylosis, herniated nucleus pulposus (HNP), trauma, tumor, reactive arthritis (RA)	68.7% neurologic improvement; 76.6% pain improvement; 93.8% fusion rate	C
DuBois et al[23]	2007	Retrospective, case control	Degenerative disease	Odom ratings similar; dynamic group with 16% nonunion vs 5% rigid	B
Saphier et al[27]	2007	Prospective cohort	Degenerative disease	Fusion rates and patient satisfaction similar	C
Goldberg et al[28]	2007	Retrospective, case control	2-level degenerative disease	Fusion rates similar between rigid and dynamic plates	B
Pitzen et al[21]	2009	Prospective, randomized, controlled	Trauma, single- and 2-level DDD	Fusion rates similar; dynamic lost 3.6° lordosis vs static plate; VAS/ODI similar	A
Nunley et al[22]	2009	Prospective, randomized, controlled	Degenerative disease	Fusion rates similar; single-level procedure VAS/ODI scores similar; double level VAS/ODI improved with dynamic plate	A

properties of a semirigid fixation system have not been determined.

PEEK is a polymer that has been studied in spinal fusion. The material properties of PEEK make it popular for several reasons. It is a biocompatible polymer, with excellent strength, virtually no reactivity, and it is radiolucent (**Fig. 3**).[38] Ponnappan and colleagues[33] compared the biomechanical properties of 5.5-mm PEEK rods with those of 5.5-mm titanium rods for single-level posterolateral fusion (PLF), and when paired with posterior lumbar interbody fusion (PLIF). They found no significant difference in stiffness between the PLF constructs in flexion/extension, lateral bending, or axial rotation. The PLIF constructs were significantly stiffer than the PLF constructs in all 3 planes. Again, there were no differences between the titanium and PEEK constructs with PLIF. The PEEK constructs with interbody graft did show increased load sharing with the interbody graft compared with the titanium posterior instrumentation. A PEEK posterior rod with an interbody graft may improve load sharing with interbody fusions, thereby encouraging compression of the interbody graft. The PEEK constructs also showed reduced stress at the pedicle screw to bone interface, which may reduce the risk of pedicle screw loosening. The ability to visualize the fusion mass is also a noted advantage of PEEK rods. There are no published clinical data that support improved outcome regarding fusion rates or screw loosening.

Nitinol is a nickel and titanium memory alloy. The flexibility and rigidity of the alloy vary with the temperature of the surrounding environment. These material properties allow the alloy to be contoured at room temperatures, and to return to a precontoured position at body temperature. The Bio-Flex System (Bio-Spine; Korea) consists of titanium pedicle screws and coiled 4-mm Nitinol rods. Kim and colleagues[36] described the use of this system in a heterogeneous cohort of patients and treatment modalities for degenerative disease of the lumbar spine. Used in combination with PLIF, the fusion rate achieved was 90%, and the overall success rate was 90.7%. The investigators reported that adjacent segment motion was increased at levels adjacent to the Bio-Flex system alone and at combined Bio-Flex/PLIF levels, and concluded that the Bio-Flex system allows for more physiologic movement at the adjacent segments. The effect of increased motion at segments adjacent to instrumented levels on degeneration will require long-term follow-up. Further evaluation of nitinol semirigid fixation will require matched comparison with rigid fixation systems.

The AccuFlex System (Globus Medical Inc; Audubon, PA, USA) is a semirigid rod designed for use with a standard pedicle screw instrumentation system. Through a proprietary technique, helical cuts are made in a 6.5-mm rod, making the rod less rigid. This system is limited to single-level use, and because the orientation of the helical

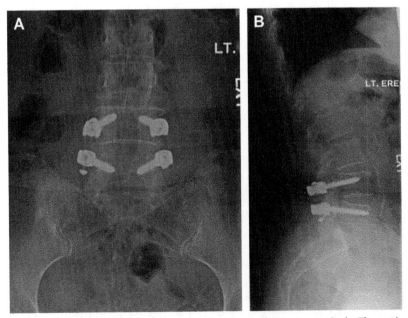

Fig. 3. Anteroposterior (A) and lateral (B) radiographs taken 3 months postoperatively. The patient is a 61-year-old woman treated for L4-L5 degenerative spondylolisthesis with L4-L5 posterior spinal fusion using PEEK rods. (*Courtesy of* Shane Burch, MD, San Francisco, CA.)

cuts is fixed, the rod is not amenable to contouring. The results for a randomized controlled trial of single-level posterior spinal fusion (PSF) with interbody fusion with standard 6.5-mm rods versus AccuFlex rods were reported by Mandigo and colleagues.[35] At 1 year of follow-up, results with respect to Short Form 36 (SF-36) scores, VAS scores, and fusion rates did not differ between the 2 groups. The investigators were careful to note that more follow-up is needed to determine whether rates of adjacent segment disease are different between the groups.

The Twinflex system (Eurosurgical; Beaurains, France) is a flexible system, based on 2.5-mm stainless steel rods, and pedicle screw fixation. The smaller diameter rods allow for less rigid fixation, again with the hypothesis that load sharing will allow for high fusion rates with less adjacent segment disease. A well-designed study by Korovessis and colleagues[39] compared this system with rigid and semirigid pedicle screw systems. With 15 patients per group and an average of 4 years follow-up, no differences in clinical results were observed. Three patients in the dynamic Twinflex group sustained broken implants, but fusion rates were similar within all 3 groups. Adjacent segment disease was not observed in any of the groups. These investigators concluded that, as the results were similar among all groups, no clear recommendations may be made. In this case, further follow-up and cost analyses may help clarify the usefulness of these different instrumentation systems.

The Dynesys (Centerpulse/Zimmer, Winterthur, Switzerland) system is marketed as a fusion device, despite a lack of peer-reviewed reports available to assess its utility for this purpose. Dynamic stabilization of the spine without fusion remains a controversial strategy in the management of spinal disorders. The Dynesys dynamic stabilization system is a pedicle screw–based construct, with polyethylene terephthalate cords and polyurethane sleeves bridging the pedicle screws. The cord acts to stabilize the motion segment in flexion, whereas the sleeve acts to stabilize in extension, and this effect has been shown in cadaveric studies.[40,41] As with other dynamic devices, the intention of instrumentation with this device is to minimize the effect of stabilization on the adjacent segments, thereby lowering the incidence of adjacent segment disease. The designers of the device reported good results at 3-year follow-up in 73 patients undergoing dynamic stabilization for degenerative disease with the Dynesys system.[42] Eleven patients suffered "complications related to the implant," with 2 requiring reoperation. An additional 11 patients underwent additional surgery for persistent pain or adjacent segment disease. Despite these high complication rates (30%), the trial investigators concluded that the implant was a success for management of degenerative lumbar disease. Statistically significant changes were observed in VAS and Oswestry Disability Index (ODI) scores. Comparison with a matched cohort treated with rigid stabilization will be useful in an assessment of the Dynesys system for treatment of degenerative lumbar pathology without fusion.

Dynesys instrumentation has been reported with variable outcomes in recent publications. Beastall and colleagues[43] used positional magnetic resonance imaging (MRI) to compare instrumented segment and adjacent segment motion following rigid instrumentation and Dynesys instrumentation. The investigators confirmed the motion-sparing and stabilizing properties of Dynesys compared with rigid instrumentation, as the dynamic stabilization group had a greater, although still restricted, range of motion (ROM) at the instrumented level. Their results, however, were opposite to the in vitro results of Schmoelz and colleagues,[41] as extension was limited, rather than flexion. With only 9 months follow-up, Beastall and colleagues[43] did confirm that adjacent segment motion was unchanged following Dynesys instrumentation. However, this same group found MRI evidence of progressive degenerative disease at Dynesys instrumented levels and at adjacent levels. Whether this is a result of the natural history of degenerative disease, as suggested by Hilibrand and colleagues[6] in the cervical spine, or a result of the intervention is unknown and will require further follow-up. In a separate investigation comparing adjacent segment ROM after Dynesys and rigid instrumentation, Cakir and colleagues[44] found no difference in ROM from the preoperative and postoperative periods. They conclude that Dynesys shows no beneficial effect on the adjacent segment.

Patient-based outcome measures are an important tool for assessing device efficacy, and represent the most important measure of implant performance. Grob and colleagues[45] presented results in their report of 2 years follow-up of a heterogeneous group of lumbar degenerative disease patients who underwent dynamic stabilization. Their results show that only 50% of patients reported that the procedure helped or helped a lot. When comparing their results with historical controls treated with fusion procedures for similar indications, these results were inferior. They note that 19% of the patients studied required reoperation within the short follow-up period. They conclude that there is no evidence to support that dynamic stabilization is superior to fusion regarding clinical outcome or need for revision surgery at the same or an adjacent level. Clinical results were also reported by Bothmann and colleagues[46] in a review of 40 patients with an average of 16 months follow-up. Subjective improvements in pain and quality of life were reported in 73% of the patients studied. These clinical improvements were similar to results from traditional fusion surgery. The investigators conclude that dynamic stabilization alone is not a successful procedure, and stabilization should be accompanied by decompression of the neural elements. An alarming reoperation rate of 27.5% was reported, with 17.5% of patients suffering from loosening of the pedicle screws. Implant loosening and high reoperation rates are important limitations in the published efficacy of dynamic stabilization systems without fusion.

Conclusion

Semirigid instrumentation of the spine may be applied with the intent to fuse the spine, or to stabilize the affected motion segment without fusion. The optimal rigidity of a posterior instrumentation system for fusion remains undetermined. Preclinical data support semirigid fixation improving the load on the interbody graft. There is little evidence that semirigid fixation may improve PLF rates (**Table 2**). Long-term follow-up of the effect of semirigid fixation on adjacent segment pathology will permit an evaluation of the technology as a strategy for preventing adjacent segment degeneration.

TRAUMA

Dynamic stabilization of the spine may be a useful strategy in protecting the neural elements and facilitating fracture healing in trauma affecting the spine. With advances in minimally invasive spinal surgery (MIS) techniques and a clinical interest in limiting fusion levels, the applications and indications for dynamic stabilization has grown in thoracolumbar trauma.[47,48] Arthrodesis of the spine, including segments above and below the affected levels, is an important and useful technique for the treatment of fractures and dislocations of the spine. Open anterior, posterior, and combined anterior and posterior approaches may involve significant blood loss and associated morbidity. Motion-sparing techniques in thoracolumbar trauma include anterior column stabilization with percutaneous vertebral augmentation, and limited instrumentation without fusion for temporary internal stabilization. In the latter case, pedicle

Table 2
Review of evidence for dynamic lumbar spine fusion constructs

Authors	Year	Study Design	Indications	Results	Grade of Evidence
Kim et al[36]	2007	Retrospective case series; Nitinol implants	Heterogeneous	VAS/ODI improved; no change adjacent segment ROM	C
Mandigo et al[35]	2007	Retrospective case/control Accuflex/rigid rod	Axial back pain	Similar VAS/SF-12 scores; similar fusion rates	C
Korovessis et al[39]	2004	Prospective randomized comparative cohorts TwinFlex/semirigid/rigid	Degenerative lumbar stenosis	VAS/SF-36 scores similar; fusion rates similar; no adjacent segment disease	A

screw and rod instrumentation is used as an internal splint for the injured level, and may be removed after soft tissue and bony healing has occurred.[49]

Thoracolumbar trauma requires extension of stabilization above and below affected segments in posterior-only approaches due to high rates of implant failure and progressive kyphosis in short fusions without anterior column support.[50,51] Stabilization of the anterior column with percutaneous vertebral augmentation may be a useful and effective technique to stabilize the spine and permit effective limited short segment posterior-only fusion.[52,53] Vertebral augmentation of the fractured level without fusion may be a useful technique for preservation of motion in thoracolumbar fractures. Costa and colleagues[54] described the use of vertebroplasty and kyphoplasty alone for the management of thoracolumbar burst fractures. Further study of the role of vertebral augmentation as a technique for anterior column stabilization will require long-term follow-up of clinical and radiographic outcome and comparison with a control group.

MIS techniques may have a role in stabilizing the spine with or without an associated fusion. Stabilization of the fractured or dislocated segments with internal fixation without fusion may permit healing of bone and ligament structures, while preserving adjacent segment motion. The published evidence to support the use of MIS techniques for internal splinting without fusion in thoracolumbar trauma is limited.[47–49] Assaker[47] has written an excellent review of the techniques available to the surgeon, and reports his indications and results with these techniques. Rampersaud and colleagues[48] and Dekutoski[55] have described excellent results in 4 patients undergoing temporary internal fixation following thoracolumbar trauma, and have shown that temporary internal stabilization may be performed safely (Fig. 4). In each of these patients the hardware was removed after the tissues had healed. An important limitation on the use of posterior fixation without fusion is that a second surgery will always be indicated, before implant failure due to fatigue. Fracture settling was observed in the burst fracture patients, but no increase in kyphosis was noticed during the follow-up period.[48] Wild and colleagues[49] compared techniques of temporary internal fixation for thoracolumbar trauma with conventional open surgery and fusion. The investigators reported on 10 patients undergoing MIS stabilization without fusion and 11 patients treated with conventional open surgery and fusion. Significant differences were noted between measures of

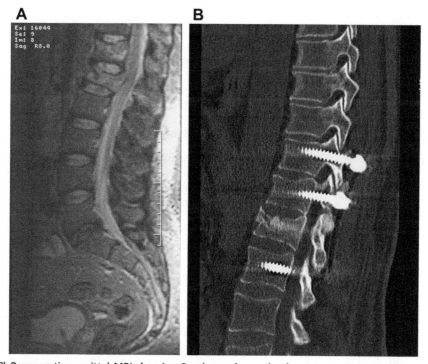

Fig. 4. (*A, B*) Preoperative sagittal MRI showing 3 column thoracolumbar trauma. Postoperative computerized tomography scan showing percutaneous stabilization from T11 to L2. Removal of hardware was planned at the time of stabilization. (*Courtesy of* Mark Dekutoski, MD, Rochester, MN.)

Table 3
Review of motion-sparing spine trauma evidence

Authors	Year	Study Design	Indications	Results	Grade of Evidence
Wild et al[49]	2007	Retrospective case/control Open/MIS	AO type A fracture	Less blood loss with MIS; SF-36 scores, Hannover spine scores similar; correction similar	B
Dai et al[58]	2009	Prospective, randomized, controlled Fusion/nonfusion	Denis type B	Frankel score, American Spinal Injury Association (ASIA) score, VAS, SF-36 scores similar; sagittal alignment similar	A
Toyone et al[57]	2006	Prospective case series Vertebral augmentation with temporary internal fixation	Thoracolumbar burst	67% without back pain; 100% with 1 grade ASIA improvement; lumbar lordosis restored; no implant failure	B

intraoperative and postoperative blood loss; MIS surgery had less blood loss. No significant differences were found in follow-up SF-36 and Hannover spine scores. Implant removal was performed an average of 10 months after the index procedure in the patients treated with an MIS approach without fusion. When removal of hardware is not planned, the hardware failure rate has been shown to be similar (14%) to cases performed with fusion.[56] Toyone and colleagues[57] reported excellent radiographic and subjective results in a group of 15 patients treated with temporary short segment fixation accompanied by vertebral body grafting for thoracolumbar burst fractures. The highest level of evidence to support rigid fixation without fusion for burst fractures comes from Dai and colleagues.[58] In a randomized controlled trial this group confirmed the work of the previously cited articles, with reduced perioperative blood loss and excellent subjective and objective results.

Conclusion

Vertebral augmentation with kyphoplasty and vertebroplasty are useful techniques for stabilizing the anterior column in thoracolumbar trauma, and there is good evidence to support the preservation of motion using these techniques with short segment posterior fixation with or without fusion. Internal stabilization of the spine without arthrodesis may permit bone and ligamentous healing and delayed removal of implants to permit retained motion of the segments adjacent to the fracture. Long-term follow-up of maintenance of correction and clinical outcome is required to evaluate the clinical efficacy and value of the technique (**Table 3**).

SUMMARY

Dynamic stabilization of the spine has applications in cervical and lumbar degenerative disease and in thoracolumbar trauma. The evidence for dynamic stabilization of the spine as an adjunct to fusion is limited. In the cervical spine, the use of dynamic plates provides clinical results similar to rigid plates. The limitation of dynamic cervical plates is the risk of adjacent-level ossification and segmental kyphosis. There is little evidence to support the use of dynamic cervical plates instead of rigid anterior cervical fixation.

Evidence to support the use of dynamic constructs for fusion in the lumbar spine is also limited with little clinical or preclinical evidence. Semirigid fixation in the lumbar spine may lead to improved loading of the interbody graft, but the effect of semirigid fixation on PLF rates has not yet been studied. The optimal mechanical properties of semirigid fixation devices to promote effective arthrodesis have not been determined. Fusion rates, implant loosening, and failure are significant concerns that limit the adoption of current devices. Dynamic stabilization of the lumbar spine without arthrodesis is most thoroughly studied with the Dynesys device. Although some early series have shown excellent midterm results for this, the authors are unable to recommend this procedure without further follow-up, as implant-related complications, including loosening, and the need for revision surgery in some series have been high.

Vertebral augmentation with vertebroplasty and kyphoplasty is a useful technique for anterior column support and effectively permits the use of shorter posterior fusion. The temporary use of rigid fixation in the management of burst fractures without excessive loss of height or canal compromise has been shown to be effective in level I studies, and the authors do recommend this intervention as an alternative to long segment or combined fusion. The need to remove implants at a second surgery is a significant limitation of the technique and requires discussion with the patient, and patient compliance. In patients with more severe kyphotic deformity and dislocation of spinal segments, arthrodesis is a more reliable approach to prevent late deformity and recurrence of displacement.

A brief synopsis of articles limited to human subjects only are listed in with grades of evidence. The current cost of health care, and spine care in particular, has highlighted the need for high-quality evidence for interventions for spinal pathology.[59] To provide convincing evidence for the effectiveness of these interventions, studies must focus on validated subjective and objective results, so that the relative values of these interventions may be calculated. Prospective randomized trials are the gold standard for investigating surgical interventions and alternative devices, and efforts to produce these studies should be supported. Lower-level studies including prospective clinical trials with appropriate outcomes and case-control studies remain an important source of information. An evidence-based approach to the management of spinal disorders will require ongoing assessment of clinical outcomes and comparison of effectiveness between alternatives.

REFERENCES

1. Gibson JN, Waddell G. Surgery for degenerative lumbar spondylosis: updated Cochrane Review. Spine (Phila Pa 1976) 2005;30(20):2312–20.

2. Feighan JE, Stevenson S, Emery SE. Biologic and biomechanic evaluation of posterior lumbar fusion in the rabbit. The effect of fixation rigidity. Spine (Phila Pa 1976) 1995;20(14):1561–7.

3. Zdeblick TA. A prospective, randomized study of lumbar fusion. Preliminary results. Spine (Phila Pa 1976) 1993;18(8):983–91.

4. Zdeblick TA, Shirado O, McAfee PC, et al. Anterior spinal fixation after lumbar corpectomy. A study in dogs. J Bone Joint Surg Am 1991;73(4):527–34.

5. Cheh G, Bridwell KH, Lenke LG, et al. Adjacent segment disease following lumbar/thoracolumbar fusion with pedicle screw instrumentation: a minimum 5-year follow-up. Spine (Phila Pa 1976) 2007;32(20):2253–7.

6. Hilibrand AS, Carlson GD, Palumbo MA, et al. Radiculopathy and myelopathy at segments adjacent to the site of a previous anterior cervical arthrodesis. J Bone Joint Surg Am 1999;81(4):519–28.

7. Park P, Garton HJ, Gala VC, et al. Adjacent segment disease after lumbar or lumbosacral fusion: review of the literature. Spine (Phila Pa 1976) 2004;29(17): 1938–44.

8. Eck JC, Humphreys SC, Lim TH, et al. Biomechanical study on the effect of cervical spine fusion on adjacent-level intradiscal pressure and segmental motion. Spine 2002;27(22):2431–4.

9. Goodship AE, Kenwright J. The influence of induced micromovement upon the healing of experimental tibial fractures. J Bone Joint Surg Br 1985;67(4): 650–5.

10. Cunningham BW, Gordon JD, Dmitriev AE, et al. Biomechanical evaluation of total disc replacement arthroplasty: an in vitro human cadaveric model. Spine (Phila Pa 1976) 2003;28(20):S110–7.

11. Robertson JT, Papadopoulos SM, Traynelis VC. Assessment of adjacent-segment disease in patients treated with cervical fusion or arthroplasty: a prospective 2-year study. J Neurosurg Spine 2005;3(6):417–23.

12. Oxford centre for evidence-based medicine - levels of evidence. 2009. Available at: http://www.cebm.net/index.aspx?o=1025. Accessed January 21, 2010.

13. Geisler FH, Caspar W, Pitzen T, et al. Reoperation in patients after anterior cervical plate stabilization in degenerative disease. Spine (Phila Pa 1976) 1998; 23(8):911–20.

14. Wang JC, McDonough PW, Endow KK, et al. Increased fusion rates with cervical plating for two-level anterior cervical discectomy and fusion. Spine (Phila Pa 1976) 2000;25(1):41–5.

15. Wang JC, McDonough PW, Kanim LE, et al. Increased fusion rates with cervical plating for three-level anterior cervical discectomy and fusion. Spine (Phila Pa 1976) 2001;26(6):643–6 [discussion: 646–7].

16. Rhee JM, Riew KD. Dynamic anterior cervical plates. J Am Acad Orthop Surg 2007;15(11):640–6.

17. Reidy D, Finkelstein J, Nagpurkar A, et al. Cervical spine loading characteristics in a cadaveric C5 corpectomy model using a static and dynamic plate. J Spinal Disord Tech 2004;17(2):117–22.

18. Brodke DS, Klimo P Jr, Bachus KN, et al. Anterior cervical fixation: analysis of load-sharing and stability with use of static and dynamic plates. J Bone Joint Surg Am 2006;88(7):1566–73.

19. Epstein NE. Anterior cervical dynamic ABC plating with single level corpectomy and fusion in forty-two patients. Spinal Cord 2003;41(3):153–8.

20. Casha S, Fehlings MG. Clinical and radiological evaluation of the Codman semiconstrained load-sharing anterior cervical plate: prospective multi-center trial and independent blinded evaluation of outcome. J Neurosurg 2003;99(3 Suppl):264–70.

21. Pitzen TR, Chrobok J, Stulik J, et al. Implant complications, fusion, loss of lordosis, and outcome after anterior cervical plating with dynamic or rigid plates: two-year results of a multi-centric, randomized, controlled study. Spine (Phila Pa 1976) 2009;34(7): 641–6.

22. Nunley PD, Jawahar A, Kerr EJ 3rd, et al. Choice of plate may affect outcomes for single versus multilevel ACDF: results of a prospective randomized single-blind trial. Spine J 2009;9(2):121–7.

23. DuBois CM, Bolt PM, Todd AG, et al. Static versus dynamic plating for multilevel anterior cervical discectomy and fusion. Spine J 2007;7(2):188–93.

24. Mahring M. [Segment changes in the cervical spine following cervical spondylodeses of unstable injuries]. Unfallchirurgie 1988;14(5):247–58 [in German].

25. Yang JY, Song HS, Lee M, et al. Adjacent level ossification development after anterior cervical fusion without plate fixation. Spine (Phila Pa 1976) 2009; 34(1):30–3.

26. Park JB, Cho YS, Riew KD. Development of adjacent-level ossification in patients with an anterior cervical plate. J Bone Joint Surg Am 2005;87(3):558–63.

27. Saphier PS, Arginteanu MS, Moore FM, et al. Stress-shielding compared with load-sharing anterior cervical plate fixation: a clinical and radiographic prospective analysis of 50 patients. J Neurosurg Spine 2007;6(5):391–7.

28. Goldberg G, Albert TJ, Vaccaro AR, et al. Short-term comparison of cervical fusion with static and dynamic plating using computerized motion analysis. Spine (Phila Pa 1976) 2007;32(13):E371–5.

29. Bono CM, Lee CK. Critical analysis of trends in fusion for degenerative disc disease over the past 20 years: influence of technique on fusion rate and clinical outcome. Spine (Phila Pa 1976) 2004;29(4): 455–63 [discussion: Z5].

30. Bridwell KH, Sedgewick TA, O'Brien MF, et al. The role of fusion and instrumentation in the treatment of degenerative spondylolisthesis with spinal stenosis. J Spinal Disord 1993;6(6):461–72.

31. Mackay JS, Mackay M, Herkowitz HN, et al. 1997 Volvo Award winner in clinical studies. Degenerative lumbar spondylolisthesis with spinal stenosis: a prospective, randomized study comparing decompressive laminectomy and arthrodesis with and without spinal instrumentation. Spine (Phila Pa 1976) 1997;22(24):2807–12.

32. Ghiselli G, Wang JC, Bhatia NN, et al. Adjacent segment degeneration in the lumbar spine. J Bone Joint Surg Am 2004;86(7):1497–503.

33. Ponnappan RK, Serhan H, Zarda B, et al. Biomechanical evaluation and comparison of polyetheretherketone rod system to traditional titanium rod fixation. Spine J 2009;9(3):263–7.

34. Bono CM, Kadaba M, Vaccaro AR. Posterior pedicle fixation-based dynamic stabilization devices for the treatment of degenerative diseases of the lumbar spine. J Spinal Disord Tech 2009; 22(5):376–83.

35. Mandigo CE, Sampath P, Kaiser MG. Posterior dynamic stabilization of the lumbar spine: pedicle based stabilization with the AccuFlex rod system. Neurosurg Focus 2007;22(1):E9.

36. Kim YS, Zhang HY, Moon BJ, et al. Nitinol spring rod dynamic stabilization system and Nitinol memory loops in surgical treatment for lumbar disc disorders: short-term follow up. Neurosurg Focus 2007; 22(1):E10.

37. Schwarzenbach O, Berlemann U, Stoll TM, et al. Posterior dynamic stabilization systems: DYNESYS. Orthop Clin North Am 2005;36(3):363–72.

38. Kurtz SM, Devine JN. PEEK biomaterials in trauma, orthopedic, and spinal implants. Biomaterials 2007; 28(32):4845–69.

39. Korovessis P, Papazisis Z, Koureas G, et al. Rigid, semirigid versus dynamic instrumentation for degenerative lumbar spinal stenosis: a correlative radiological and clinical analysis of short-term results. Spine (Phila Pa 1976) 2004;29(7):735–42.

40. Schulte TL, Hurschler C, Haversath M, et al. The effect of dynamic, semi-rigid implants on the range of motion of lumbar motion segments after decompression. Eur Spine J 2008;17(8):1057–65.

41. Schmoelz W, Huber JF, Nydegger T, et al. Dynamic stabilization of the lumbar spine and its effects on adjacent segments: an in vitro experiment. J Spinal Disord Tech 2003;16(4):418–23.

42. Stoll TM, Dubois G, Schwarzenbach O. The dynamic neutralization system for the spine: a multi-center study of a novel non-fusion system. Eur Spine J 2002;11(Suppl 2):S170–8.

43. Beastall J, Karadimas E, Siddiqui M, et al. The Dynesys lumbar spinal stabilization system: a preliminary report on positional magnetic resonance imaging findings. Spine (Phila Pa 1976) 2007;32(6):685–90.

44. Cakir B, Carazzo C, Schmidt R, et al. Adjacent segment mobility after rigid and semirigid

instrumentation of the lumbar spine. Spine (Phila Pa 1976) 2009;34(12):1287–91.

45. Grob D, Benini A, Junge A, et al. Clinical experience with the Dynesys semirigid fixation system for the lumbar spine: surgical and patient-oriented outcome in 50 cases after an average of 2 years. Spine (Phila Pa 1976) 2005;30(3):324–31.

46. Bothmann M, Kast E, Boldt GJ, et al. Dynesys fixation for lumbar spine degeneration. Neurosurg Rev 2008;31(2):189–96.

47. Assaker R. Minimal access spinal technologies: state-of-the-art, indications, and techniques. Joint Bone Spine 2004;71(6):459–69.

48. Rampersaud YR, Annand N, Dekutoski MB. Use of minimally invasive surgical techniques in the management of thoracolumbar trauma: current concepts. Spine (Phila Pa 1976) 2006;31(11 Suppl):S96–102 [discussion: S104].

49. Wild MH, Glees M, Plieschnegger C, et al. Five-year follow-up examination after purely minimally invasive posterior stabilization of thoracolumbar fractures: a comparison of minimally invasive percutaneously and conventionally open treated patients. Arch Orthop Trauma Surg 2007;127(5):335–43.

50. McLain RF, Burkus JK, Benson DR. Segmental instrumentation for thoracic and thoracolumbar fractures: prospective analysis of construct survival and five-year follow-up. Spine J 2001;1(5):310–23.

51. Parker JW, Lane JR, Karaikovic EE, et al. Successful short-segment instrumentation and fusion for thoracolumbar spine fractures: a consecutive 41/2-year series. Spine (Phila Pa 1976) 2000;25(9):1157–70.

52. Korovessis P, Repantis T, Petsinis G, et al. Direct reduction of thoracolumbar burst fractures by means of balloon kyphoplasty with calcium phosphate and stabilization with pedicle-screw instrumentation and fusion. Spine (Phila Pa 1976) 2008; 33(4):E100–8.

53. Marco RA, Kushwaha VP. Thoracolumbar burst fractures treated with posterior decompression and pedicle screw instrumentation supplemented with balloon-assisted vertebroplasty and calcium phosphate reconstruction. J Bone Joint Surg Am 2009; 91(1):20–8.

54. Costa F, Ortolina A, Cardia A, et al. Efficacy of treatment with percutaneous vertebroplasty and kyphoplasty for traumatic fracture of thoracolumbar junction. J Neurosurg Sci 2009;53(1):13–7.

55. Dekutoski MB. Thoracolumbar fracture management with selective fusion and instrumentation removal in IMAST. Hong Kong, 2008.

56. Sanderson PL, Fraser RD, Hall DJ, et al. Short segment fixation of thoracolumbar burst fractures without fusion. Eur Spine J 1999;8(6):495–500.

57. Toyone T, Tanaka T, Kato D, et al. The treatment of acute thoracolumbar burst fractures with transpedicular intracorporeal hydroxyapatite grafting following indirect reduction and pedicle screw fixation: a prospective study. Spine (Phila Pa 1976) 2006;31(7):E208–14.

58. Dai LY, Jiang LS, Jiang SD. Posterior short-segment fixation with or without fusion for thoracolumbar burst fractures. A five to seven-year prospective randomized study. J Bone Joint Surg Am 2009; 91(5):1033–41.

59. Martin BI, Deyo RA, Mirza SK, et al. Expenditures and health status among adults with back and neck problems. JAMA 2008;299(6):656–64.

Contemporary Management of Symptomatic Lumbar Disc Herniations

Kolawole A. Jegede, BS, Anthony Ndu, MD,
Jonathan N. Grauer, MD*

KEYWORDS

• Symptomatic lumbar disc herniations
• Contemporary management • Lumbar related symptoms

Lumbar disc herniations are common clinical entities that may cause lumbar-related symptoms. The spectrum of treatment options is geared toward a patient's clinical presentation and ranges from nothing to surgical intervention. Many lumbar disc herniations cause no significant symptoms. In studies of asymptomatic individuals who have never experienced lumbar-related symptoms, 30% have been reported to have major abnormality on magnetic resonance imaging.[1] The mainstay of treatment of patients with symptomatic disc herniations is accepted to be nonoperative (as long as there are no acute or progressive neurologic deficits); this includes medications, physical therapy, and potentially lumbar injection.[2–4] For patients with symptomatic disc herniations who fail to respond appropriately to conservative measures, surgical intervention may be considered. For this population, lumbar discectomy is considered to be a good option.

LUMBAR DISCECTOMY

Discectomy is the most common operation performed in the United States for patients who are experiencing lumbar-related symptoms.[5] Nonetheless, despite the wide acceptance of discectomy as a treatment option for symptomatic lumbar disc herniation, there has been a paucity of level I evidence supporting the effectiveness of

this surgery compared with nonoperative care.[6] Significant regional variation in discectomy rates in the United States and lower international rates have also raised questions about when these surgeries should be performed.[7]

Several studies have compared surgical and nonoperative treatment, but small sample sizes, study design limitations, and failure to plan for high crossover rates limit the strength of these studies. Between the years of 1983 and 2007 there were 4 randomized controlled trials (RCTs) comparing operative care with more conservative management, not including the well-publicized Spine Patient Outcomes Research Trial (SPORT).[5,8–12]

Weber[9] performed a controlled, prospective study with 10 years of follow-up. Of the 280 patients enrolled in this study, 126 were randomized to either surgery or physical therapy. The others were not randomized and had surgery or nonoperative treatment. The group randomized to surgery had statistically better outcomes after 1 year. After 4 years, however, although the surgery outcomes were still better, this difference was no longer statistically significant.

Buttermann[12] conducted a prospective, randomized study comparing epidural steroid injection (ESI) with discectomy for treatment of lumbar disc herniation. One hundred patients who had failed noninvasive therapy for 6 weeks were randomly

Department of Orthopaedics and Rehabilitation, Yale University School of Medicine, PO Box 208071, New Haven, CT 06510-8071, USA
* Corresponding author.
E-mail address: jonathan.grauer@yale.edu

Orthop Clin N Am 41 (2010) 217–224
doi:10.1016/j.ocl.2010.01.003
0030-5898/10/$ – see front matter © 2010 Elsevier Inc. All rights reserved.

assigned to receive ESI or discectomy. This study found that discectomy patients had more rapid improvement in their symptoms. The investigators stated that ESI was not as effective as surgery in reducing symptoms in those with large herniations.

Osterman and colleagues[8] conducted a prospective, randomized study comparing physical therapy with discectomy for treatment of lumber disc herniation. Fifty-six patients who had radiating back pain below the knee for 6 to 12 weeks were randomized to receive either isometric physical therapy or discectomy. Patients were followed for 2 years and at final follow-up the study found no clinically significant difference between the groups in terms of leg pain intensity and other secondary outcomes. These investigators proposed discectomy provided only some short-term benefit.

Another study by Peul and colleagues[11] was a prospective, randomized study comparing nonsurgical treatment with discectomy for the treatment of lumbar disc herniation. Two hundred and eighty subjects were followed for a year and the investigators found that the 2 groups had similar outcomes at 1 year, but those who underwent surgery had faster rates of recovery and self-perceived pain.

These studies together contribute significant information about the outcomes that can be expected from lumbar discectomy. For an outcome measure, Weber[9] used a patient-described 4-tier descriptive scale (poor, fair, good, excellent). The 3 other more recently published studies by Osterman and colleagues,[8] Peul and colleagues,[13] and Butterman[12] used more common general and disease-specific health quality surveys, and clinical examination. Each of these studies had 1 year follow-up, except for Weber's, in which long-term follow-up to 10 years after surgery was included.

Crossover rates were an issue for each of these RCTs. The crossover from nonsurgical treatment group to the surgical treatment group ranged from 34.7%[9] to 54%,[12] with the average being 42.6%. In each of these studies, a smaller number of patients crossed over from the surgical treatment group to the nonsurgical treatment group, with an average of 21.4%.[10]

Two of the 4 studies used an intent-to-treat (ITT) analysis.[8,9] Weber used an ITT analysis but also used tables to show the treatment assigned and the treatment received. However, in the primary analysis these investigators left out the 34.7% of patients who crossed over to the surgical group. Osterman and colleagues used an ITT and an as-treated analysis but the as-treated analysis was not reported in detail.

The results of these lumbar disc herniation RCTs were variable when compared with each other.

The general observed trend was that early outcomes were improved with surgical intervention, but longer-term outcomes were more similar when comparing nonoperative and surgical management.

SPORT TRIAL

The SPORT trial was a federally funded, multicenter, prospective, randomized, controlled study assessing the efficacy of surgery versus nonsurgical treatment of lumbar intervertebral disc herniation. This large undertaking took more than 7 years to complete and was published in the *Journal of the American Medical Association* in 2006.[5] Despite the tremendous amount of work and resources that were put into this research study, the primary investigators were unable to make a definitive statement about the advantage of any 1 treatment type, largely because of issues with study group crossover.[5,14]

The main goal of this trial was to evaluate the efficacy of surgery versus nonoperative treatment of lumbar disc herniation. Patients were enrolled over a 4-year period from 13 multidisciplinary spine clinics in 11 US states. Investigators screened 2720 patients and 1991 were found eligible. Of these 1991 patients, 1244 enrolled in the trial, 501 agreeing to be randomized, and 743 enrolled in an observational arm of the study.[15] The primary outcomes measures used in this study were changes in the Medical Outcomes Study Health Survey bodily pain and physical function scales and the modified Oswestry Disability Index for a 2-year period.

The study reported that the ITT analysis showed significant improvement in all measured outcomes in both treatment groups. The investigators concluded by stating that because of high crossover rates from both groups, no direct comparison between surgical and nonsurgical management was warranted based on the ITT analysis.[5] The a priori null hypothesis of no difference between surgical and nonsurgical treatments was thus unable to be ruled out.[14,16]

The issues noted with this high-profile study have led to much scrutiny.[8,16–18] Despite a clear statement by the study investigators that direct comparisons between the 2 treatments would not be valid, many have interpreted the results to suggest equivalence between surgery and nonsurgical care for patients with lumbar disc herniations.[5] The error in these statements was most likely caused by the reader interpreting the treatment groups in the SPORT trial as the treatment received. However, because of the ITT analysis and a high crossover rate, the nonoperative group contained many patients who did have surgery. The surgical benefits for those patients who crossed over into the surgery treatment group were allocated to nonoperative care and clearly biased the results toward the null hypothesis.[14]

SPORT STUDY HYPOTHESIS

The formation of a reasonable and clinical relevant study hypothesis is extremely important for the success of a prospective, randomized clinical trial.[19] The only hypothesis that can be assessed by this type of study is one that is stated before the study takes place. The stated a priori hypothesis of the SPORT study was simply to determine if there was no difference between surgical and nonsurgical management in patients with lumbar disc herniations. The dichotomous hypothesis was intended to give an answer to whether surgery was superior to nonoperative care.

This simplified hypothesis proved problematic in many ways. The stated hypothesis implied that lumbar disc herniation is a uniform condition, with surgery and nonoperative care as the competing treatments.[10] In current practice, surgical and nonsurgical treatments for lumbar disc herniations are not thought of as competing or transposable options but rather treatments along a spectrum of care. Further, lumbar disc herniation is a heterogeneous condition with differences in pain severity, neurologic impairment, natural history, and treatment response.[14]

The main goals in treatment of patients presenting with this heterogeneous condition are alleviating pain and returning function with as little risk as possible.[20–22] Hence, almost all patients who present with painful lumbar disc herniation without acute or progressive neurologic deficit begin treatment with nonsurgical approaches. Most surgeons would be hesitant to offer surgical treatment to a patient who has pain for a short duration or who is actively improving. This situation makes it difficult to randomize patients to one of these otherwise staged treatment options.[14,22]

SPORT STUDY POPULATION

Randomization to surgical versus nonsurgical treatments is challenging. Based on this, despite multiple centers collecting patients over a significant period of time, it is difficult to fully power a study. This complication has contributed to concern that the SPORT study could have inadvertently biased toward the null hypothesis[14] and may have created a situation in which the study would fail to recognize a difference between surgical and nonsurgical treatment groups when one exists (type II error).

As mentioned earlier, patients presenting with symptomatic lumbar disc herniation would likely initially be treated with nonsurgical management. Those who were presenting with mild or improving symptoms would continue treatment with less invasive measures. Almost 20% of patients randomized to receive surgery in the RCT group had self-reported mild/moderate symptoms that were improving.[15] There is class II evidence that patients with mild symptoms who undergo surgery usually do not have a significant treatment benefit compared with nonsurgical treatment.[21] In current clinical practice these patients may not have undergone surgery. However, whether or not the 20% of mildly affected patients in the RCT crossed over to nonoperative treatment or had surgery, their treatment response to surgery would be associated with the surgical group. The inclusion of this patient population underestimated the effects of surgery in the study compared with what would be encountered in clinical practice.

The underestimation of the benefits of surgery also holds true for severely symptomatic patients assigned to the nonsurgical treatment group. Severely affected patients are known to receive the highest benefit from surgery[21] and many of the patients assigned to the nonsurgical group crossed over in this study. All the benefits associated with surgery as a result of this high crossover were credited to the nonsurgical treatment group because of the ITT analysis. In both instances the effect was to underestimate the advantages of surgery and overestimate the advantages of nonsurgical management in relation to what would occur in current clinical practice.

Because surgery is known to benefit those with severe symptoms, and in the current study patients identified to have severe symptoms were less likely to enroll in the SPORT RCT, this would also have the effect of underestimating the effects of surgery in relation to what would be observed in current clinical practice. Analyzing the observational cohort population in SPORT shows that 75% of these patients had severe symptoms, which was significantly worse than the average symptom severity in the RCT population, and they chose to undergo surgery.[15] The other 25% of this cohort was made up of patients with mild disease who mostly initially chose nonsurgical treatment. Patients who had severe symptoms were more likely to refuse to enter the randomization group and again this underestimated the effects of surgery. The overall effect of 3 of 4 patients choosing not to be randomized causes further underestimation of the true benefit

Table 1
Studies comparing nonsurgical with surgical treatment of lumbar disc herniation

Study	Treatment	Level of Evidence	Clinical Outcomes	Pros	Cons
Weinstein et al[5]	Physical therapy versus discectomy	Level 1	The ITT analysis was reported as no clinical or statistical difference between the 2 treatment groups at any time point. The as-treated analysis strongly favored surgery at all time points during 2 years	Largest study comparing operative versus nonoperative treatment of lumbar disc herniation. The multisite prospective randomized clinical control trial enrolled more than 1244 patients	Study had a significant number of crossovers. Investigators stated that no conclusions about comparability about the treatments under study can be made because of the ITT analysis
Weber[9]	Inpatient physical therapy versus discectomy	Level I	At 1 year, surgery had better outcomes that were statistically significant in the ITT analysis and the analysis excluding crossovers	Patients in this study were followed for up to 10 years, which is the longest for any study of this time. Study had the lowest crossover rate of any study of its kind	The primary statistical analysis excludes the patients who crossed over from nonoperative to operative management
Buttermann[12]	ESI versus discectomy	Level I	ESI was not so effective as discectomy with regard to reducing symptoms and disability associated with a large herniation of the lumbar disc	Despite many prior studies of ESI in nonoperatively treated patients this was the first RCT to directly compare the effects of ESI versus discectomy	The study had a significant number of crossovers into the surgery group (54%), which may have substantially affected any results. There was no clear indication if the study included crossovers in the surgical group

Osterman et al[8]	Isometric physical therapy versus discectomy	Level 1	Reported no significant difference between the surgical group and nonsurgical group up to the 2-year follow-up. ITT and as-treated analysis showed similar results	Study was randomized and had acceptable rate of follow-up. Presented data in ITT and as-treated analysis	Study had a small side and did not account for crossovers. Study experienced a 39.3% crossover rate. An as-treated analysis was performed but the details were not reported
Peul et al[11]	6 months of continual nonsurgical treatment versus early discectomy	Level I	Patients who underwent early discectomy had less severe symptoms and less disability early on, but by year 1 the differences disappeared	Second largest study comparing nonsurgical treatment with surgical intervention. Nine-center prospective study, RCT	Study did not account for crossovers and experienced a 38.7% crossover into the surgery group. ITT analysis was performed without accounting for these crossovers
Atlas et al[21]	Open discectomy versus nonoperative treatment	Level II	Surgically treated patients were on average more symptomatic at entry. Surgically treated patients with sciatica reported substantially greater improvement at 1-year follow-up	Study reported a large number of patients with a small size. Patient and their physician were allowed to make treatment decisions, which potentially made the study more clinically relevant	All patients and physicians were limited to 1 geographic area. Lumbar spine surgery rates vary by geographic area. No randomization took place in this study

of surgery within the SPORT RCT compared with what would be seen in current clinical practice.[5,14]

HIGH CROSSOVER RATE

With a power of 0.85 the authors expected to see a 10-point difference in the surveys of patient health with the sample size chosen. However, based on the literature on lumbar disc herniation, a significant crossover rate should have been expected.[8,9,11–13] The large crossover rate causes a reduction in the difference observed between the 2 treatment groups. Patients with severe symptoms assigned to nonsurgical treatment were more likely to cross over to the surgery group, whereas patients with mild symptoms assigned to the surgical group were likely to cross over to the nonsurgical group.

This high crossover rate significantly decreased the power of the study and hence the ability of the study to detect any difference between the treatments groups, even if one existed. The failure of the investigators to include any crossover rate in their study design or power calculation severely weakened SPORT. With a crossover rate around 45% in the SPORT RCT the effective power of the study was only 7%, compared with the 85% reported.[14] The clinical appropriateness and cost-effectiveness of this study may have been questioned if any consideration of crossover were made before the study began.

NO STRATIFICATION OF KNOWN PROGNOSTIC FACTORS

Early studies have found a strong correlation between pretreatment symptom severity and treatment outcomes in regards to lumbar disc herniation. The Main Lumbar Spine Study[21] showed that patients who reported serious neurologic symptoms had better response to surgery than nonoperative management that was clinically and statistically significant. Surgery was found to be less effective compared with nonsurgical treatment in those who presented with mild symptoms. The intensity of presenting symptoms was an available prognostic factor but is difficult to control for in an RCT.

The inability to stratify by these and other prognostic factors and instead blindly randomize patients may decrease the clinical relevance of a study and make data difficult to interpret. The randomization without thought of the prognostic factors masks the beneficial effects of surgery in patients with severe symptoms by combining them with patients with mild symptoms, who are known not to benefit from more invasive procedures.

DISCUSSION

RCTs are considered to be the most powerful studies in medical literature.[23,24] Such studies lead to what is referred to as level I evidence and usually command great respect from the scientific community. However, the difficulties faced by SPORT and the other RCT discussed reveal that there are limitations to such studies.[25,26]

RCTs that attempt to compare surgical versus nonsurgical treatments are particularly difficult to design and perform.[10] Patient compliance, randomization, and blinding investigators and patients are challenging or impossible. Further, varying severity of presenting symptoms affects the treatment options and treatment response.[5]

The goal of the investigators of SPORT and the other RCTs investigating lumbar disc herniations was to take the results from their representative sample population and to generalize them to anyone with lumbar disc herniation. This is a challenging objective. Not only were the patients already those presenting for surgical evaluation, but those who agree to enroll in RCTs may be different from those who refuse to participate.

The investigators compared the RCT patient cohort with the nonrandomized observational cohort.[15] Although the study reported no statistically significant differences between the 2 groups, a closer look revealed substantial differences in measurements of pain, disability, and perceptions of their own health state. The observational group was essentially divided into 2 distinct populations composed mostly of those with severe symptoms that were significantly worse than the average seen in the RCT cohort. The differences seen in these groups could have significantly affected the response treatment. It could also be assumed that similar differences could have been noted in the 719 patients who refused to participate in the study completely. That there are substantial differences between those who decide to participate in a randomized clinical trial and those who do not shows that any results reported may not be generalizable to the population.

ITT analysis is the statistical tool that protects randomization. Use of ITT analysis makes the assumption that the treatment that the patient initially assigned is the treatment that the patient received at some time point.[27] As the rate of crossover increases, the effects of randomization diminish. Crossover from treatment groups decreases the only desired difference that the investigators would want to see between the randomly assigned groups, which is the treatment that is received.

If no crossover occurs between 2 randomly assigned treatment groups then the assumed difference in outcome can be validly related to the treatment received. On the other hand, if half the patients in a particular treatment group cross over into the opposite group it will be impossible to detect a difference. It is not surprising that Weinstein and colleagues[5] reported no difference between treatments, with more than 40% of patients crossing over at the 2-year time point.

SPORT was 1 of the few RCTs assessing the benefits of surgery in lumbar disc herniation to state an a priori power calculation but did not take into account the crossover rate that ended up being observed. The investigators stated that with a power of 0.85 they would expect to see a 10-point difference in the 36-item Short Form Health Survey (SF-36) scale used and a similar effect size in the Oswestry Disability Index with the sample size they chose.[5] This calculation was assuming that there would be a 100% compliance with the assigned treatment. When taking into account the crossover rate seen in the SPORT trial, the power of the study was calculated to be 0.07.[14] If the investigators had assumed a crossover rate of at least 25% based on prior studies[9,12] the power of the SPORT RCT would still be only 0.32.[14]

Despite the efforts of a large multicenter RCT, SPORT was unable to provide valid data on the effect size of the 2 treatments studied, because the crossover rates were so high. Because of this crossover rate and many other factors, the power that is usually associated with RCTs was lost in this study. Despite the overwhelming preference given to RCTs there is no clear statement that observational studies and RCTs produce consistently dissimilar results.[25,26] All the RCTs of lumbar disc herniation treatment performed over the last 2 decades consistently had high crossover rates and were not able to definitively answer important questions about patient care.[10] These recurring issues raise the question if it is possible to conduct a valid and quality RCT of treatment outcomes for lumbar disc herniation (**Table 1**).

REFERENCES

1. Boden SD, Davis DO, Dina TS, et al. Abnormal magnetic-resonance scans of the lumbar spine in asymptomatic subjects. A prospective investigation. J Bone Joint Surg Am 1990;72:403–8.
2. Mathews JA, Mills SB, Jenkins VM, et al. Back pain and sciatica: controlled trials of manipulation, traction, sclerosant and epidural injections. Br J Rheumatol 1987;26:416–23.
3. Derby R, Kine G, Saal JA, et al. Response to steroid and duration of radicular pain as predictors of surgical outcome. Spine (Phila Pa 1976) 1992;17:S176–83.
4. Riew KD, Yin Y, Gilula L, et al. The effect of nerve-root injections on the need for operative treatment of lumbar radicular pain. A prospective, randomized, controlled, double-blind study. J Bone Joint Surg Am 2000;82:1589–93.
5. Weinstein JN, Tosteson TD, Lurie JD, et al. Surgical vs nonoperative treatment for lumbar disk herniation: the Spine Patient Outcomes Research Trial (SPORT): a randomized trial. JAMA 2006;296:2441–50.
6. Rhee JM, Schaufele M, Abdu WA. Radiculopathy and the herniated lumbar disc. Controversies regarding pathophysiology and management. J Bone Joint Surg Am 2006;88:2070–80.
7. Weinstein JN, Bronner KK, Morgan TS, et al. Trends and geographic variations in major surgery for degenerative diseases of the hip, knee, and spine. Spine 2006;31:2707–14. Suppl Web Exclusives: VAR81–9.
8. Osterman H, Seitsalo S, Karppinen J, et al. Effectiveness of microdiscectomy for lumbar disc herniation - a randomized controlled trial with 2 years of follow-up. Spine 2006;31:2409–14.
9. Weber H. Lumbar disc herniation. A controlled, prospective study with ten years of observation. Spine (Phila Pa 1976) 1983;8:131–40.
10. Anderson PA, McCormick PC, Angevine PD. Randomized controlled trials of the treatment of lumbar disk herniation: 1983–2007. J Am Acad Orthop Surg 2008;16:566–73.
11. Peul WC, van Houwelingen HC, van den Hout WB, et al. Surgery versus prolonged conservative treatment for sciatica. N Engl J Med 2007;356:2245–56.
12. Buttermann GR. Treatment of lumbar disc herniation: epidural steroid injection compared with discectomy. A prospective, randomized study. J Bone Joint Surg Am 2004;86:670–9.
13. Peul WC, van den Hout WB, Brand R, et al. Prolonged conservative care versus early surgery in patients with sciatica caused by lumbar disc herniation: two year results of a randomised controlled trial. BMJ 2008;336:1355–8.
14. McCormick PC. The Spine Patient Outcomes Research Trial results for lumbar disc herniation: a critical review. J Neurosurg Spine 2007;6:513–20.
15. Weinstein JN, Lurie JD, Tosteson TD, et al. Surgical vs nonoperative treatment for lumbar disk herniation: the Spine Patient Outcomes Research Trial (SPORT) observational cohort. JAMA 2006;296:2451–9.

16. Angevine PD, McCormick PC. Wrong science: the SPORT trial and its potential impact on neurosurgery. Clin Neurosurg 2004;51:120–5.

17. McCormick PC. The need for outcome studies. What are we doing in neurosurgery? Clin Neurosurg 2001; 48:193–203.

18. McCormick PC. Spine Patient Outcome Research Trial (SPORT): multi-center randomized clinical trial of surgical and non-surgical approaches to the treatment of low back pain. Spine J 2003;3:417–9.

19. McPeek B, Mosteller F, McKneally M. Randomized clinical trials in surgery. Int J Technol Assess Health Care 1989;5:317–32.

20. Deyo RA, Loeser JD, Bigos SJ. Herniated lumbar intervertebral disk. Ann Intern Med 1990;112:598–603.

21. Atlas SJ, Deyo RA, Keller RB, et al. The Maine Lumbar Spine Study, Part II. 1-year outcomes of surgical and nonsurgical management of sciatica. Spine (Phila Pa 1976) 1996;21:1777–86.

22. Hoffman RM, Wheeler KJ, Deyo RA. Surgery for herniated lumbar discs: a literature synthesis. J Gen Intern Med 1993;8:487–96.

23. Louis TA, Shapiro SH. Critical issues in the conduct and interpretation of clinical trials. Annu Rev Public Health 1983;4:25–46.

24. Moher D, Dulberg CS, Wells GA. Statistical power, sample size, and their reporting in randomized controlled trials. JAMA 1994;272:122–4.

25. Benson K, Hartz AJ. A comparison of observational studies and randomized, controlled trials. N Engl J Med 2000;342:1878–86.

26. Concato J, Shah N, Horwitz RI. Randomized, controlled trials, observational studies, and the hierarchy of research designs. N Engl J Med 2000;342: 1887–92.

27. Little R, Yau L. Intent-to-treat analysis for longitudinal studies with drop-outs. Biometrics 1996;52: 1324–33.

Clavicle Fractures in 2010: Sling/Swathe or Open Reduction and Internal Fixation?

Michael D. McKee, MD, FRCS(C)

KEYWORDS

• Clavicle • Fixation • Randomized trials • Evidence-based
• Comparative studies • Review

Clavicle fractures are common, and they comprise close to 3% of all fractures seen in fracture clinics. Midshaft fractures account for approximately 80% of all clavicle fractures and are the focus of this article. Distal clavicle fractures are next most common, consisting of 15% of clavicle fractures, and medial third fractures are the least common, making up 5% of injuries. Distal third and medial third fractures are distinct entities and have a separate set of features requiring different approaches to imaging, diagnosis, and treatment compared with middle third fractures.

Traditionally, even widely displaced midshaft clavicle fractures have been treated nonoperatively based on several large studies that demonstrated excellent functional outcome with various methods of closed reduction and nonoperative treatment. In the past, most of the controversy surrounded the optimal method (if any) of nonoperative treatment, with various investigators supporting simple sling treatment, figure-of-eight bandaging, or other types of external support. Operative methods were deemed to have a high complication rate and little role in the primary treatment of fractures. The nonunion rate after nonoperative treatment was described as being approximately 1%, even in widely displaced fractures, and malunion was described as being of radiographic interest only.[1–5]

However, recent studies have reported significantly different outcomes with regard to completely displaced fractures of the clavicle. Studies that have used patient-based outcome measures (as opposed to the more traditional surgeon-based or radiographic outcomes) have described an unsatisfactory outcome rate of 25% to 31%.[5–15] Multiple comprehensive, prospective studies have clearly shown the nonunion rate in this setting to be up to 21%, exponentially higher than previously reported. In addition, a significant number of patients with malunited fractures have ongoing symptomatology with orthopedic, neurologic, and functional cosmetic deficits in a characteristic pattern; it would appear that clavicular malunion is a distinct clinical entity.

There are multiple potential explanations for the increased rate of poor outcome including survival of critically injured trauma patients with more severe fracture patterns, increased patient expectations of having a normal shoulder after injury, comprehensive follow-up (including patient-oriented outcome measures), and excluding children (with their inherently good prognosis) from analysis.

These findings spurred further investigation into comparative studies examining the role of primary operative fixation (usually consisting of compression plating or intramedullary nailing) in the treatment of displaced midshaft fractures of the clavicle. These comparative investigations including those examining different methods of closed treatment, operative versus nonoperative treatment, and different

The devices that are the subject of this article are FDA approved.
Nothing of benefit was received with regard to this article.
Division of Orthopaedics, Department of Surgery, St Michael's Hospital and the University of Toronto, 55 Queen Street East, Suite 800, Toronto, ON M5C 1R6, Canada
E-mail address: mckeem@smh.toronto.on.ca

Orthop Clin N Am 41 (2010) 225–231
doi:10.1016/j.ocl.2009.12.005

methods of operative fixation are the focus of this evidence-based medicine article.

TREATMENT OPTIONS

Although a variety of treatment options have been described for the treatment of midshaft fractures of the clavicle, they can be summarized in 3 main types: nonoperative, open reduction and internal fixation with a plate, and intramedullary pin fixation (through either an open or closed reduction technique). These options, and the articles supporting them, are described in the following sections.

Nonoperative

Nonoperative care is the treatment of choice for most fractures of the clavicle shaft, especially those that are minimally displaced or undisplaced or those that occur in elderly, ill, noncompliant, or sedentary individuals in whom the risk of surgical intervention is too high or the potential benefit is too low. There have been multiple different techniques and devices described to obtain and maintain a satisfactory nonoperative reduction of a displaced midshaft fracture of the clavicle. However, there is little or no convincing evidence that any significant improvement can be made to the original position of the fracture in most cases, and one must typically accept the displacement seen on injury films. Although some temporary improvement in alignment may well occur with various techniques, such as the figure-of-eight bandage (traditionally popular in North America), there is little evidence that this device can maintain a closed reduction of a displaced clavicle fracture.

Currently, immobilization with a simple sling until the patient is comfortable enough to begin a gradual return to preinjury activities is the commonest nonoperative treatment choice. A randomized trial by Andersen and colleagues[15] examined the functional and radiographic results after the use of a figure-of-eight bandage versus a simple sling for the treatment of displaced midshaft fractures of the clavicle. They found no significant difference between the 2 groups at final follow-up in either radiographic or functional outcome. Also, patients preferred the sling (2/27 dissatisfied with sling versus 9/34 dissatisfied with figure-of-eight bandage, $P = .09$). For this reason, it is reasonable to consider nonoperative treatment groups in comparative studies as one homogenous group in terms of outcome, despite the fact that there may be some differences in the type of nonoperative therapy used.

The results of nonoperative treatment were previously thought to be satisfactory in most cases, but modern studies with patient-based outcome measures have revealed significant deficits. Hill and colleagues[7] reported a high degree of residual patient dissatisfaction after nonoperative treatment of displaced midshaft clavicle fractures using a patient-based outcome tool. They found a nonunion rate of 15%, and overall 31% of patients were dissatisfied with their outcome. In a study examining 225 clavicle fractures, Nordqvist and colleagues[8] described good results after long-term follow-up with 185 good, 39 fair, and only 1 poor result. It should be noted that in the subcategory of displaced, comminuted fractures 27% of patients rated their shoulder as fair and this corresponds to the dissatisfied group (31%) in Hill's study. Nowak and colleagues[6] reported that 46% of 208 patients treated nonoperatively had shoulder sequelae at 9- to 10-year follow-up. In a study from the fracture group in Edinburgh, Robinson and colleagues[4] reported on a prospective, consecutive series of 868 patients with clavicle fractures, 581 of whom had a midshaft diaphyseal fracture, and described a nonunion rate of 21% in displaced comminuted midshaft fractures. Brinker and colleagues[5] analyzed the data from that article and suggested a nonunion rate of 33% for displaced comminuted fractures in men.

What is clear from these articles is that a significant percentage of young active patients with displaced midshaft clavicle fractures treated nonoperatively will develop symptomatic nonunion or malunion. These patients complain of a short, droopy, ptotic, asymmetric shoulder with orthopedic (weakness, rapid fatiguability), neurologic (thoracic outlet), and functional cosmetic (difficulty wearing backpacks, straps, etc) symptomatology.

Open Reduction and Plate Fixation

Open reduction and plate fixation of displaced midshaft fractures of the clavicle using modern precontoured implants and techniques has been well described with a high degree of success and low complication rate.[12–14] Older reports of operative fixation that described a high failure rate and an unacceptable level of complications were plagued by selection bias (only the worst, comminuted, open fractures received surgery), poor soft-tissue handling, and fixation methods (cerclage wires or short, weak plates) that could reasonably be described as suboptimal by modern standards.[1–3] Modern studies have reported significantly improved results after plate fixation. Smith and colleagues[16] reported union in all of the 30 cases treated in this manner in a prospective trial, Collinge and colleagues[17] reported union in 39 of 42 cases treated with anterior/inferior plating, and Poigenfürst and colleagues[12] reported excellent results in

122 consecutive cases treated with superior plating. The operative group in the randomized clinical trial performed by the Canadian Orthopaedic Trauma Society (COTS) reported only 2 nonunions out of 62 cases treated with plate fixation. Although there are disadvantages with this technique including plate prominence (and subsequent hardware removal) and potential wound complications from the dissection required, in most modern series the incidence is low. In addition, precontoured anatomic plates are now available that minimize local irritation and decrease the need for hardware removal. A careful 2-layer (deltotrapezial fascia/platysma muscle and skin/subcutaneous tissue) closure can decrease the incidence and morbidity of potential infection. Although it remains controversial, antero-inferior placement of the plate has been advocated as a means of decreasing local irritation (as well as avoiding neurovascular structures while drilling).[17]

Intramedullary Pin Fixation

Various retrospective reviews describe various methods of intramedullary pinning of the clavicle.[18–23] The main intrinsic difficulty is that of trying to perform intramedullary fixation of a curved bone with a straight intramedullary device. The theoretical advantages of this technique are many and include minimal soft tissue dissection at the fracture site, less soft tissue prominence of the hardware, and a reduced refracture rate when compared with plate fixation. If the pin does need to be removed, it can be done through a small incision with minimal dissection, often under local anesthetic. Chuang and colleagues[23] reported success in 30 of 31 midshaft clavicle fractures treated with closed reduction and an intramedullary screw technique. Boehme and colleagues[19] reported similar results in a series that included both fractures and nonunions. In addition, newer techniques describe insertion of smaller diameter elastic or flexible nails using a completely closed method. The fracture is reduced under image intensifier control and the pin is passed through a medial entry portal, across the fracture site, and impacted laterally.[18,24] Disadvantages of this technique include difficulty in controlling shortening and rotation at the fracture site, especially if there is significant comminution. This may explain the inconsistent results seen with this technique when compared with nonoperative care (see later section).

COMPARATIVE STUDIES

While there are many retrospective, single-arm studies that describe results after the treatment of various types of clavicle fractures, there are only relatively few prospective or randomized trials published. This section details high-quality comparative studies on a specific subgroup of injuries: completely displaced midshaft fractures of the clavicle in young (16–60 years of age) healthy patients.

Sling Versus Figure-of-Eight Bandage

There is evidence (2 randomized trials and multiple retrospective reviews) that a sling is as effective as a figure-of-eight bandage in immobilizing fractures of the clavicle and is favored by patients.[15,25] There is no conclusively proven difference in radiographic or functional outcome regardless of the method of nonoperative treatment chosen. Lenza and colleagues,[25] in a Cochrane Database Review of 234 nonoperatively treated patients from 3 randomized controlled trials, concluded that there was no evidence to support one nonoperative technique over another. For this reason the authors' current treatment of choice for displaced midshaft fractures of the clavicle is a simple sling for comfort, followed by early range of motion exercise as pain diminishes.

Plate Fixation Versus Nonoperative Care

A multicenter, prospective, randomized clinical trial on this topic was performed by the COTS. One hundred thirty-two patients with completely displaced fractures of the midshaft clavicle were randomized to nonoperative (sling) or operative (open reduction and plate fixation) treatment.[26] Although, as with most young male trauma populations, a significant number of patients were lost to follow-up, 111 patients were analyzed at a year after injury. Analysis of both surgeon- and patient-based outcome scores revealed significantly improved Constant and disabilities of the arm, shoulder and hand (DASH) scores in the operative group (**Figs. 1** and **2**) with fewer nonunions (2/62 vs 7/49, $P = .042$) and symptomatic malunions (0/62 vs 9/49, $P = .001$). Complications in the operative group included hardware removal in 5 cases and local infections in 3 cases. These were treated with a single repeat operative procedure. In a similar study, which has been presented but not published, Smith and colleagues[16] performed a prospective randomized trial comparing primary plate fixation with nonoperative care (sling) in 102 patients. This study was also complicated by a high rate of patients lost to follow-up, but the investigators found that open reduction and plate fixation resulted in union of all the 30 cases studied, whereas the nonoperative group had 12 nonunions in 35 cases ($P = .001$). They concluded that plate fixation was safe,

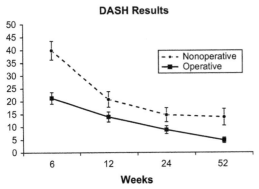

Fig. 1. Acute displaced midshaft fractures of the clavicle. Graphical analysis of mean Constant shoulder scores in the operative plate fixation group versus nonoperative group at 6 weeks, 12 weeks, 24 weeks, and 52 weeks follow-up. Values are statistically improved for the operative group at each time point (P<.01 for all). (*Adapted from* COTS study; Canadian Orthopaedic Trauma Society. Nonoperative treatment compared with plate fixation of displaced midshaft clavicle fractures. A multicenter, randomized clinical trial. J Bone Joint Surg Am 2007;89:7; with permission.)

effective, and superior to nonoperative care with regard to preventing nonunion and improving patient function. They reported a 30% rate of hardware removal. It is important to note that both these studies were performed before the availability of anatomic precontoured plates.

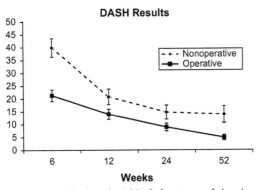

Fig. 2. Acute displaced midshaft fractures of the clavicle. Graphical analysis of mean DASH scores in the operative plate fixation group versus non-operative groups at 6 weeks, 12 weeks, 24 weeks, and 52 weeks follow-up. The DASH is a disability score in whicha perfect extremity would typically score 0 (mean values for a normal population are in the 4–8 range). Values are worse in the nonoperative group at each time point (6 week P<.01, 12 week P = .04, 24 week P = .05, 52 week P<.01). (*Adapted from* COTS study; Canadian Orthopaedic Trauma Society. Nonoperative treatment compared with plate fixation of displaced midshaft clavicle fractures. A multicenter, randomized clinical trial. J Bone Joint Surg Am 2007;89:8; with permission.)

Based on these studies there is evidence that primary plate fixation of completely displaced midshaft fractures of the clavicle improves patient outcome and reduces the rate of nonunion and symptomatic malunion when compared with nonoperative care. This information is used when making a decision with the patient as to the optimal treatment method for their fracture.

Intramedullary Pin Fixation Versus Nonoperative Treatment

A randomized prospective trial performed in a US military population compared nonoperative care with intramedullary fixation (modified Hagie pin) of displaced clavicle fractures. There was no statistically or clinically significant difference in shoulder outcome scores at 1 year (operative 93 vs nonoperative 98).[22] Also, complications were significantly higher in the operative group, including nonunion, refracture, infection, and pin prominence. However, the high rate of loss of reduction in the operative group (47%, leading to pin prominence as the fracture site shortened) indicates that fixation was suboptimal. An earlier retrospective study compared nonoperative (figure-of-eight bandage) with operative (intramedullary pin fixation) treatment in an Asian civilian population.[21] The investigators reported no significant differences in shoulder scores (nonoperative 85 vs operative 83) at final review. The operative group had several complications including 8 infections, 3 refractures, 2 hardware failures, and 2 nonunions (14 of 40 patients, 35%). This technique using an open reduction with a large diameter pin does not appear to be as consistently successful as plate fixation. This may be due to several as-yet unclear factors including patient selection (size, compliance), fracture patterns (comminution), or surgery (technique, implant type).

In a randomized trial of 60 patients with completely displaced midshaft clavicle fractures, Smekal and colleagues[24] compared a different type of intramedullary device, a smaller diameter elastic nail, with the nonoperative (sling) treatment. The investigators described a technique in which the fracture was reduced and the nail was inserted under radiographic control in a closed fashion in most cases. They reported superior outcomes in the operative group with better DASH and Constant scores at multiple time points up to and including 24 months after injury. There were 3 nonunions and 2 symptomatic malunions requiring correction in the nonoperatively treated group compared with no such complication in the group treated with a pin. However, there was pin protrusion in 7 patients and 2 required revision surgery.

Table 1
Meta-analysis of nonoperative treatment, intramedullary pinning, and plate fixation for displaced midshaft fractures of the clavicle (Published 1975–2005)

Treatment	Nonunion (%)	Infections (%, Total)	Infections (%, Deep)	Fixation Failures (%)
Non-operative, N=159	15.1	0	0	0
Plating, n=460	2.2	4.6	2.4	2.2
Intramedullary pinning, n=152	2.0	6.6	0	3.9

Data from Zlowodzki M, Zelle BA, Cole PA, et al. Treatment of mid-shaft clavicle fractures: systemic review of 2144 fractures. J Orthop Trauma 2005;19(7):504–8.

The authors concluded that their operative technique resulted in a decreased delayed and nonunion rate, resulted in a faster return to function, and provided better long-term functional outcome compared with nonoperative treatment.

Although intramedullary pin fixation remains promising, at the present time the results in comparative studies are too inconsistent to make any definite conclusions about one treatment over another.

Plate Fixation Versus Intramedullary Nailing

Because no comparative prospective or randomized study has been published comparing the outcome of plating with intramedullary nailing of

Table 2
Comparative trials of operative versus nonoperative treatment of displaced midshaft fractures of the clavicle

Author/ Year	Design	LOE	Study Recommendations	Pros	Cons
COTS 2007	RCT	A	ORIF with plate superior to sling (superior DASH, Constant scores)	Good design, multicenter, large number of patients	More patients in nonoperative group lost to follow-up
Smith et al, 2000	RCT	A	ORIF with plate superior to sling	Randomized design	Presented, never published in full due to poor follow-up rate
Grassi et al, 2001	Retrospective, comparative	B	Nonoperative care superior to intramedullary nailing	Large study	Retrospective, unusually high surgical complication rate
Judd et al, 2009	RCT	A	Sling equal to Hagie pin, higher complications in pin group	Randomized design	Small numbers (57), single center
Smekal et al, 2009	RCT	A	Elastic intramedullary nailing superior to sling	Good design, randomized	Surgical technique new and unproven

Abbreviations: DASH, disabilities of the arm, shoulder, and hand; LOE, level of evidence; ORIF, open reduction and internal fixation; RCT, randomized clinical trial.

Table 3
Recommendations for the optimal treatment of displaced midshaft fractures of the clavicle

Statement	Grade of Recommendation	References
Young active patients with completely displaced midshaft fractures of the clavicle will have superior results with primary fracture fixation.	B	14,16,24,26
Antero-inferior plating may reduce the risk of symptomatic hardware compared with superior plating.	C	17
There is no difference in outcome between a regular sling and a figure-of-eight bandage when nonoperative treatment is selected.	B	15,25
There is no difference in outcome between plating and intramedullary nailing of displaced midshaft clavicle fractures.	I	10,12,14,18–21,23
Factors associated with poor outcome after nonoperative treatment of displaced midshaft clavicle fractures include shortening and increasing fracture comminution.	A	4–7,9,14,16

displaced clavicular fractures, no specific recommendation can be made. Indirect inference can be made from the fact that 2 separate randomized trials show advantages of plate fixation over nonoperative care,[16,26] whereas similar studies with intramedullary nailing as the operative technique are inconsistent.[20–22] The theoretical advantages of intramedullary nailing (decreased soft tissue dissection, reduced hardware prominence, reduced refracture rate) may not outweigh the difficulties in maintaining length and rotation of the fracture (drawbacks of any unlocked intramedullary device). The only information currently available is an unpublished retrospective review with small numbers (17 patients per group), which suggested superiority of intramedullary pinning over plate fixation or nonoperative care for displaced midshaft clavicle fractures.[20]

Meta-analyses on Clavicle Fracture Treatment

A meta-analysis of available data from articles on midshaft clavicle fractures published between 1975 and 2005 has been published.[14] This meta-analysis contains information regarding all treated clavicle fractures, but for the purpose of this article data regarding displaced fractures are specifically assessed. A nonunion rate of 15.1% was observed after nonoperative care of such injuries, whereas the nonunion rate for similar fractures treated with plate fixation was 2.2%. The nonunion rate for fractures treated with intramedullary pinning was 2%. Therefore, plating a displaced fracture of the clavicle resulted in a decrease in the nonunion rate from 15.1% to 2.2% when

compared with nonoperative treatment; this represents a relative risk reduction of 86%, (95% CI = 71%–93%). A meta-analysis performed by the Cochrane Database Review examined 3 trials that compared a sling with a figure-of-eight bandage[2] or low-intensity pulsed ultrasound versus placebo[1] in the treatment of displaced midshaft fractures. There were methodological problems with each study, and no significant differences in functional or other outcome could be shown. The investigators concluded that, at the present time, there is no evidence to support the superiority of one nonoperative technique over another (**Tables 1–3**).[25]

SUMMARY

The topic of this article is completely displaced midshaft fractures, which represent a specific subset of clavicle injuries. Prospective and randomized studies using thorough and complete assessment measures show that the rate of unsatisfactory outcome after nonoperative treatment is significant—a 15% to 20% rate of nonunion and a 20% to 25% rate of symptomatic malunion. Fracture factors that portend a poor outcome include displacement or shortening of more than 2 cm and fracture comminution. If nonoperative treatment is chosen, sling immobilization followed by early range of motion is recommended. Primary plate fixation of displaced midshaft clavicle fractures improves outcome, results in earlier return to function, and reduces the nonunion and symptomatic malunion rate significantly compared with nonoperative treatment. Results from randomized studies using intramedullary pinning are inconsistent at present, and it remains to be determined if the theoretical advantages of this technique will translate into clinical practice. The information from these high-quality studies can be used to decide on the optimal treatment method for each individual patient.

REFERENCES

1. Rowe CR. An atlas of anatomy and treatment of mid-clavicular fractures. Clin Orthop Relat Res 1968;58: 29–42.
2. Crenshaw AH. Fractures of the shoulder girdle, arm and forearm. In: Crenshaw AH, editor. Campbell's operative orthopaedics. 8th edition. St. Louis (MO): Mosby-Yearbook Inc; 1992. p. 989–95.
3. Neer CS. Nonunion of the clavicle. JAMA 1960;172: 1006–11.
4. Robinson CM, Court-Brown CM, McQueen MM, et al. Estimating the risk of nonunion following non-operative treatment of a clavicle fracture. J Bone Joint Surg Am 2004;86(7):1359–65.
5. Brinker MR, Edwards TB, O'Connor DP. Estimating the risk of nonunion following nonoperative treat-ment of a clavicular fracture. [letter to the editor]. J Bone Joint Surg Am 2005;87(3):677–8.
6. Nowak J, Holgersson M, Larsson S. Can we predict long-term sequelae after fractures of the clavicle based on initial findings? A prospective study with nine to ten years follow-up. J Shoulder Elbow Surg 2004;13(5):479–86.
7. Hill JM, McGuire MH, Crosby LA. Closed treatment of displaced middle-third fractures of the clavicle gives poor results. J Bone Joint Surg Br 1997; 79(4):537–41.
8. Nordqvist A, Petersson CJ, Redlund-Johnell I. Mid-clavicle fractures in adults: end result study after conservative treatment. J Orthop Trauma 1998; 12(8):572–6.
9. McKee MD, Wild LM, Schemitsch EH. Midshaft mal-unions of the clavicle. J Bone Joint Surg Am 2003; 85(5):790–7.
10. Basamania CJ. Claviculoplasty. J Shoulder Elbow Surg 1999;8(5):540 [abstracts: Seventh International Conference on Surgery of the Shoulder, 1999].
11. McKee MD, Stephen DJG, Kreder HJ, et al. Func-tional outcome following clavicle fractures in poly-trauma patients. J Trauma 2000;47(3):616.
12. Poigenfürst J, Rappold G, Fischer W. Plating of fresh clavicular fractures: results of 122 operations. Injury 1992;23(4):237–41.
13. McKee MD, Seiler JG, Jupiter JB. The application of the limited contact dynamic compression plate in the upper extremity: an analysis of 114 consecutive cases. Injury 1995;26(10):661–6.
14. Zlowodzki M, Zelle BA, Cole PA, et al. Treatment of mid-shaft clavicle fractures: systemic review of 2144 fractures. J Orthop Trauma 2005;19(7):504–8.
15. Andersen K, Jensen PO, Lauritzen J. The treatment of clavicular fractures: figure of eight bandage versus a simple sling. Acta Orthop Scand 1987;58:71–4.
16. Smith CA, Rudd J, Crosby LA. Results of operative versus non-operative treatment for 100% displaced mid-shaft clavicle. Proceedings from the 16th Annual Open Meeting of the American Shoulder and Elbow Surgeons. San Francisco, CA, March 8, 2000. p. 41.
17. Collinge C, Devinney S, Herscovici D, et al. Anterior-inferior plate fixation of middle-third fractures and nonunions of the clavicle. J Orthop Trauma 2006; 20(10):680–6.
18. Jubel A, Andermahr J, Schiffer G, et al. Elastic stable intramedullary nailing of mid-clavicular frac-tures with a titanium nail. Clin Orthop Relat Res 2003;408:279–85.
19. Boehme D, Curtis RJ, DeHaan JT, et al. Nonunion of fractures of the mid-shaft of the clavicle. Treatment with a modified Hagie intramedullary pin and autog-enous bone-grafting. J Bone Joint Surg Am 1991;73: 1219–26.
20. Sampath DS. Treatment of displaced midclavicle fractures with Rockwood pin: a comparative study. Proceedings of the 2005 AAOS Annual Meeting. Washington, DC, February 25, 2005. p. 566.
21. Grassi FA, Tajana MS, D'Angelo F. Management of midclavicular fractures: comparison between non-operative treatment and open intramedullary fixation in 80 patients. J Trauma 2001;50(6):1096–100.
22. Judd DB, Pallis MP, Smith E, et al. Acute operative stabilization versus nonoperative management of clavicle fractures. Am J Orthop 2009;38(7):341–5.
23. Chuang TY, Ho WP, Hsieh PH, et al. Closed reduc-tion and internal fixation for acute midshaft clavicular fractures using cannulated screws. J Trauma 2006; 60(6):1315–22.
24. Smekal V, Irenberger A, Struve P, et al. Elastic stable intramedullary nailing versus nonoperative treatment of displaced midshaft clavicular fractures-a random-ized, controlled, clinical trial. J Orthop Trauma 2009; 23(2):106–12.
25. Lenza M, Belloti JC, Andriolo RB, et al. Conservative interventions for treating middle third clavicle frac-tures in adolescents and adults [review]. Cochrane Database Syst Rev 2009;(2):CD007121.
26. Canadian Orthopaedic Trauma Society. Nonopera-tive treatment compared with plate fixation of dis-placed midshaft clavicle fractures. A multicenter, randomized clinical trial. J Bone Joint Surg Am 2007;89:1–10.

Lower Extremity Assessment Project (LEAP) – The Best Available Evidence on Limb-Threatening Lower Extremity Trauma

Thomas F. Higgins, MD*, Joshua B. Klatt, MD, Timothy C. Beals, MD

KEYWORDS

- Amputation • Limb salvage
- Lower extremity assessment project
- Mangled extremity

In a 1987 editorial in the *Journal of Bone and Joint Surgery*, Dr Sigvard Hansen, of Harborview Medical Center in Seattle, noted the profound physical, mental, social, and financial implications of futile attempts at limb salvage in the setting of severe lower extremity trauma.[1] He acknowledged the evolution of microvascular and external fixation techniques, which made "heroic" limb salvage procedures possible. Although for some patients the outcomes represent true progress in medicine, other patients had to go through years of repeated surgeries, infections, and bone grafting only to end up with a compromised amputation on a delayed basis. Many of these patients ended up demoralized, divorced, destitute, and drug addicted.

Dr Hansen called for the development of objective guidelines to influence clinicians' decisions about "amputation versus salvage" and concluded his article with the following: "Perhaps the best source would be a multicenter study done by members of the Orthopaedic Trauma Association. The development of such guidelines would help to provide an answer to this problem and thus allow both patients and their doctors to avoid prolonged, costly, and fruitless salvage procedures when such a course is not indicated."[1]

Subsequently, Johansen and colleagues[2] established the Mangled Extremity Severity Score (MESS) criteria in an effort to provide such a set of guidelines. This system, first published in 1990, attempted to stratify 4 variables: skeletal/soft tissue injury, limb ischemia, shock, and patient age. An analysis of retrospective and prospective study groups led to a recommendation that a MESS value greater than or equal to 7 was an indication for amputation. In the prospective portion of the analysis, this proved to be 100% accurate in predicting amputation. The weakness of this study is the self-fulfilling nature inherent in studying this algorithm on a prospective basis.

Even with such guidance, orthopedic surgeons continued to struggle with the decision of whether to amputate or salvage the severely injured lower extremity. Commonly held beliefs, including that an insensate plantar foot was an indication for amputation, were based on little or no evidence.

Given this obvious gap in the literature of the emerging subspecialty of orthopedic traumatology, a prospective longitudinal study was

Department of Orthopaedics, University of Utah, 590 Wakara Way, Salt Lake City, UT 84108, USA
* Corresponding author.
E-mail address: thomas.higgins@hsc.utah.edu

Orthop Clin N Am 41 (2010) 233–239
doi:10.1016/j.ocl.2009.12.006
0030-5898/10/$ – see front matter

undertaken at 8 level I trauma centers nationally. Ultimately headed by Ellen MacKenzie, PhD, a professor of Health Policy and Management at Johns Hopkins University, and Dr Michael Bosse, an orthopedic traumatologist at Carolinas Medical Center, the Lower Extremity Assessment Project (LEAP) study set out to answer many of the questions surrounding the decision to amputate or salvage. A National Institutes of Health–funded, multicenter, prospective observational study, the LEAP study represented a milestone in orthopedic trauma research, and perhaps in orthopedics.

The inclusion criteria for the LEAP study included the following:

1. Traumatic amputations below the distal femur
2. Gustilo grade IIIA open tibia fractures with hospital stays greater than 4 days, 2 or more limb procedures, and a high degree of nerve, muscle, or bone injury
3. Gustilo grade IIIB and IIIC open tibia fractures
4. Dysvascular injuries below the distal femur
5. Major soft tissue injuries below the distal femur, excluding the foot
6. Grade III open pilon fractures
7. Grade IIIB open ankle fractures
8. Severe open hindfoot and midfoot injuries with degloving and nerve injury.[3]

The LEAP study attempted to account for all variables in patients sustaining these injuries.[4] Surgeons caring for patients participating in the study would be permitted to carry out patient management as they saw fit. There was no set treatment algorithm to the study. The LEAP study attempted to define the characteristics of the individuals who sustained these injuries, the characteristics of their environment, the variables of the physical aspects of their injury, the secondary medical and mental conditions that arose from their injury and treatment, their ultimate functional status, and their general health.

Besides age, gender, and comorbidities, the values, beliefs, and psychological profiles of patients' were also assessed. The characteristics of their environment included their physical surroundings, their educational and economic backgrounds, and their social and work surroundings.[4] Assessing all of these aspects entailed the use of many assessment tools never previously used in orthopedic research.

In terms of evidence-based medicine, the LEAP study and the resulting publications are somewhat different from many evidence-based trials. There is no control of the therapeutic intervention. However, the data was prospectively collected, and the investigators have accumulated 7-year follow-up on most of the patients. With the 7-year follow-up data, examiners have attempted to record, as objectively as possible, all the potential variables in what is a complicated clinical situation. It seems that the existing lower extremity trauma scoring systems are not predictive of the outcome of salvage or amputation, but unfortunately the LEAP studies have not yielded a better or more accurate method for predicting optimal treatment.

In the final analysis, it has been learned that many of the patients sustaining this high degree of extremity trauma have a great number of social, economic, and personality disadvantages, even before their injury. Functional outcomes and quality of life outcomes seem more related to many of these preexisting factors than to interventions provided by the health care system, regardless of whether they underwent amputation or salvage. This fact may be distressing news to the orthopedic traumatologist, as this could mean that all of the prevarication and anxiety surrounding the treatment of these injuries have little long-term effect on the outcome. The alternative view would promote keeping these variables in mind and trying to maximize the support for those patients most in need at the time of severe lower extremity trauma.

Given the nature of the study, the levels of evidence are all level I or level II. There are no data in the orthopedic trauma literature to date to compare with the LEAP study, in terms of the breadth of the data recorded or the number of patients enrolled. From the standpoint of evidence-based medicine, this is the best information available.

Based on the inclusion criteria, 601 patients were enrolled for more than a period of 44 months at 8 centers. Initial patient characteristics data showed that 77% were male, 72% were white, and 71% were between the ages of 20 and 45 years. Of the patients, 70% had graduated from high school (compared with 86% nationally) and 25% lived below the federal poverty line (16% nationally), 38% had no health insurance (20% nationally), and there were twice as many heavy drinkers in this sample as in the population at large.[3] On personality inventories, these patients were noted to be slightly more neurotic, extroverted, and less open to new experiences than the remainder of the population. None of these characteristics appeared to have an influence on the likelihood of the affected limb that was going to be amputated or salvaged.

A 2002 LEAP publication in the New England Journal of Medicine compared the outcome of surgeries between those patients who underwent reconstruction and those who underwent primary amputation.[5] The major outcome variable examined was the Sickness Impact Profile (SIP). The SIP is a measure of self-reported health status, which relies on 136 statements of limitation in each of 12 subcategories. A low score on the scale represents a lower sickness impact and a score of greater than 10 in any area represents severe disability.

Two years after injury, there was no significant difference in the SIP scores between the group that underwent amputation and the group that underwent reconstruction (12.6 vs 11.8, $P = .53$). Even after adjusting for characteristics of the patients and of their injuries, functional outcomes were similar between the 2 groups. Self-efficacy is one of the characteristics assessed with SIP scores, and describes the confidence a subject has in his or her ability to perform specific tasks or activities.[4] A person with low self-efficacy may disengage from the coping process because they expect to fail. Self-efficacy and social support turned out to be highly predictive of outcome in the group that underwent reconstruction and the group that underwent amputation. Other predictors of a lower score on the SIP, included rehospitalization for a major complication, lower educational level, nonwhite race, poverty, lack of private health insurance, poor social support network, low self-efficacy, smoking, and the involvement of the patient in disability or compensation litigation. Patients who underwent reconstruction were more likely to have a secondary hospitalization for major complication than those who underwent amputation (47.5% vs 33.9%, $P = .002$). Two years after their injury, only 53% of those who underwent amputation had returned to work and 49% of those who underwent reconstruction had returned to work. Unfortunately, many of the predictors of poor SIP scores coincide with patient characteristics that are overrepresented in the severe lower extremity trauma population (lower educational level, poverty, and lack of health insurance).

The cohort of 161 patients who had undergone amputation above the ankle within 3 months of injury were further examined with the SIP, in an effort to determine the influence of amputation level on functional outcome.[6] The patients treated with amputations above the knee showed no significant difference in their SIP scores from those treated with amputations below the knee. Patients with through-knee amputations had worse regression-adjusted SIP scores than either above or below the knee amputees. Patients with amputations below their knee had the fastest walking speeds. The study also failed to find any link

between outcomes and the technological sophistication of the prosthetic device used by the amputees. Considering there are approximately 3500 traumatic major lower limb amputations per year in the United States, these findings offer some guidance to physicians; however, the level and the severity of the trauma is still the most likely determining factor for the level of amputation.

Another subset of the LEAP studies that attempted to evaluate the decision-making processes in amputation versus reconstruction was published in 2001.[7] This study included 556 of the LEAP study patients and evaluated them by 5 different injury severity scoring systems. The MESS, the Limb Salvage Index, the Predictive Salvage Index, the Nerve Injury, Ischemia, Soft Tissue Injury, Skeletal Injury, Shock, and Age of Patient Score, and the Hannover Fracture Scale-97 for ischemic and nonischemic limbs were assessed. Immediate amputation and amputation within a 6-month period were assessed. There were 63 immediate amputations and 86 delayed amputations.

The LEAP study did not support the usefulness of any of the examined lower extremity injury severity indices for determining limbs that require amputation and those likely to be successfully salvaged. Overall, these scores lacked sensitivity, but were in some cases specific. Scores at the time of injury were not useful in identifying patients that would eventually require amputation, but they might have some use in predicting which limbs could be successfully salvaged. This study tried to address the initial question of whether there are objective criteria that could be used for indicating amputation. Unfortunately, no established system was predictive, and no evidence-based alternative has been proposed.

Before the LEAP study, a widely held indication for amputation in case of lower extremity trauma was the absence of plantar sensation at the initial presentation. In 2005, an article by Bosse and colleagues[8] attempted to determine the long-term outcomes after treatment of those patients who present with the absence of plantar sensation. The study included 26 insensate plantar feet that were amputated, 29 insensate feet that were salvaged, and 29 matched controls from among the larger cohort of sensate limbs that were salvaged. At 2-year follow-up, normal plantar sensation was present in an equal proportion of those who initially had an insensate foot that was salvaged and in those who had a sensate foot that was salvaged (approximately 55%). Only 1 patient of the 29 of the insensate salvaged group had completely absent plantar sensation at 2-year follow-up, the others having at least some level of improvement. There were no significant differences in the SIP between any of the 3 groups. In summary, absent plantar sensation at the time of presentation did not prove to be an indication for amputation, a predictor of functional outcome, or even a predictor of eventual plantar sensation.

A separate study examined the 7 lower extremity injury severity indices, as they might be related to functional outcomes, 2 years after salvage.[9] Median SIP scores were 15.2 at 6 months and 6.0 at 24 months. None of the examined scoring systems were predictive of ultimate functional outcome or improvement in functional outcome between 6 and 24 months.

A subsequent grouping of the LEAP studies evaluated treatment variables that may have affected outcome. A 2007 article by Webb and colleagues[10] examined a subcohort of 156 patients to describe surgeon-controlled variables that may have affected union, complication, and functional outcome in severe open diaphyseal tibia fractures. It appeared that the timing of wound debridement (<6 hours vs 6–24 hours), the timing of soft tissue coverage (more or less than 3 days after injury), and the timing of bone grafting (more or less than 3 months after injury) did not seem to have any influence on infection rates, union rates, or functional outcome. Those fixed with intramedullary fixation had slightly less severe injuries than those fixed with external fixation, and understandably had lower SIP scores and fewer complications. The entire cohort did show deterioration in SIP scores between 2-year and 7-year follow-up.

The effect of smoking on fracture healing and complications was examined in a cohort of 268 patients with open tibia fracture.[11] A multivariate regression analysis examined those who had never smoked, those who had quit smoking, and those who were current smokers regarding their ability to heal the fracture within 24 months. The study also evaluated their time to union, the presence or absence of infection, and the presence or absence of osteomyelitis. Current smokers were 37% less likely to achieve union than nonsmokers, and previous smokers were 32% less likely to achieve union than nonsmokers. Current smokers were 2.2 times more likely to develop an infection and 3.7 times more likely to develop osteomyelitis than nonsmokers. Those who quit smoking were at no greater risk of infection overall, but were at 2.8 times greater risk for developing osteomyelitis. The effect of smoking on open tibia fractures has been examined previously, but the LEAP study certainly represents the largest cohort of prospectively collected data in which multivariate analysis could be used to isolate the effect of smoking.

The optimal type of flap coverage has been a source of dispute almost since the advent of microvascular free tissue transfer techniques. Pollak and colleagues[12] examined a cohort of 190 patients in the LEAP database who required flap coverage, and who had at least 6 months of follow-up. End points included short-term complications, such as wound infection, necrosis, and loss of the flap. There were 87 limbs treated with a rotational flap and 107 limbs treated with a free tissue transfer. In terms of selection bias, the group treated with free tissue transfer represented more severe injuries to the limb and the group treated with rotational flap had a significantly higher injury severity score for overall trauma. There were no significant differences with respect to overall complication rates. After controlling for other variables, a single difference in short-term complications was identified specifically in those patients with the most severe osseous injuries. Limbs that featured an Orthopaedic Trauma Association/AO type C bony injury that was treated with a rotational flap were 4.3 times more likely to have a wound complication requiring reoperation than those treated with a free flap. It would seem that the severity of the osseous injury might be predictive of injury to the surrounding soft tissues, which may diminish the success rate of rotating local tissue.

A separate study reported the overall complication rate for the groups with amputation and the groups with reconstruction at 2-year follow-up.[13] Of 149 limbs that underwent amputation during the initial hospitalization, the revision amputation rate was 5.4%. The complication rate at 3 months was 24.8% and one-third of these were wound infections. Out of 371 limb reconstructions, 3.9% required late amputation, 37.7% reported a complication by 6 months, one-quarter of which were wound infections, 23.7% had nonunion, and 7.7% had osteomyelitis. These numbers overall may best be used in counseling patients at the time of initial hospitalization. Although a few patients in such circumstances may be capable of participating in a truly informed decision, reconstruction does come with a higher rate of complication and rehospitalization than primary amputation, and 4% of reconstruction patients will end up with a late amputation.

A study by O'Toole and colleagues[14] attempted to examine the variables specific to patient satisfaction. None of the patient demographics, treatment characteristics, or injury characteristics was found to correlate with patient satisfaction. Five key outcome measures seemed to account for more than one-third of the overall variation in patient satisfaction: return to work, depression, the physical functioning component of their SIP, their self-selected walking speed, and their pain intensity. It seems that patient satisfaction is determined most significantly by function, pain, and presence or absence of depression.

An area of trauma care that traditionally receives little attention is psychological distress, and the LEAP study attempted to determine the rate of this particular comorbidity in severe lower limb injury. Forty-eight percent of patients tested positive a likely psychological disorder 3 months after injury, and this number only diminished to 42% at the 2-year mark.[15] Almost 20% reported severe phobic anxiety or depression, and all examined subscales of psychological distress tested higher than normative values. Unfortunately, only 12% and 22% of patients reported receiving any mental health services 3 months and 24 months after injury, respectively. This study clearly identified an area of trauma care with a room for improvement.

Another subset of injuries examined was knee dislocations with vascular injury, but there were only 18 patients in the LEAP cohort that met these criteria.[16] Four of the 18 limbs were amputated (22%) and a prolonged warm ischemia time was the factor most highly associated with amputation. SIP scores for successful reconstruction were 12 at 1 year and 7 at 2 years, compared with a 2-year SIP score of 16 for those who underwent amputation. Patients whose limbs were salvaged did much better, but these were presumably the less severe injuries.

One of the factors identified early on in the decision to reconstruct or amputate the severely traumatized lower extremity was the monetary cost associated with each treatment option. Limb salvage incurs the costs of an increased rate of subsequent hospitalization and subsequent operation for infection, soft tissue coverage, and union, whereas amputation bears the lifetime costs of prosthetics manufacture and repair. The LEAP study addressed this issue in a 2007 article in the *Journal of Bone and Joint Surgery*.[17] The cost calculations included initial hospitalization, subsequent hospitalization related to the injured limb, inpatient rehabilitation, outpatient doctor visits, outpatient physical and occupational therapy, and the purchase and maintenance of prosthetic devices. Lifetime costs were projected based on expected life years. When the prosthetic costs at 2 years were included, salvage averaged $81,316 and amputation averaged $91,106. Projected lifetime costs, however, were 3 times higher for the amputation group ($509,275 vs $163,282). It may be difficult to include monetary costs as a factor in the decision algorithm for salvage versus

amputation, but these are data that treating surgeons and potential patients may want to be aware of to fully appreciate the implications of treatment decisions.

Further analysis of the LEAP data yielded 3 publications looking at 7-year follow-up. Examining long-term work disability, 58% of 423 patients followed up to 7 years had returned to work at the 7-year mark (47% of amputees and 62% of reconstructions, the difference not being statistically significant).[18] However, even those patients who returned to work were judged to be, on average, limited in their ability to perform their job 20% to 25% of the time. Factors significantly associated with a higher rate of return to work included lower age, white race, higher education level, nonsmoking, average to high self-efficacy, preinjury job tenure, and absence of litigation in the case. The assessment of pain and physical function at just 3 months post injury was a significant predictor of ultimate return to work at 7 years.

In an attempt to examine the long-term persistence of disability at 7 years, telephone interviews of almost 400 patients were conducted and correlated with SIP scores.[19] At 7 years, half of the patients had a SIP score greater than or equal to 10 points which, according to the SIP index, indicates severe disability. One-third of all patients had a score typical of the general population for their age and gender. When adjusting for other factors, poor physical SIP subscores were significantly associated with both those limbs that had severe soft tissue injury without fracture in the reconstruction group and those who underwent through-knee disarticulation in the amputation group. There were no significant differences in the psychosocial outcome scores between the group that underwent amputation and the group that underwent salvage. Familiar patient characteristics were significantly associated with prolonged disability, and these included increasing age, female gender, nonwhite race, lower education level, poverty, current or previous smoking, low self-efficacy score, poor self-reported preinjury health status, and involvement with litigation over disability. With the exception of age, predictors of poor outcome at 24 months were the same at 7 years.

The prevalence of chronic pain at 7 years was also reported.[20] Only 23% of the LEAP study population was pain-free at 84 months, compared with 42.3% of the general population. In terms of the severity of their chronic pain on a graded scale, scores reported for the LEAP patients were similar to the primary care migraine headache population and the chronic back pain population. Significant early predictors of chronic pain were less than high school level education, less than college education, low self-efficacy, and high levels of alcohol consumption. Those patients who continued to be treated with narcotic medication 3 months post discharge had lower levels of chronic pain at the 84-month mark.

Some aspects of the LEAP study also examined the role of physical therapy in recovery.[21] Patients with amputation and reconstruction used comparable amounts of physical therapy services. The percentage of patients with a perceived need for physical therapy services but receiving no therapy increased over the course of 2-year follow-up, reaching a rate of 68% at 2 years. Risk factors for not receiving therapy included lack of private health insurance, increased pain, lower level of education, lower level of fitness at the time of injury, being a smoker, and presence of a severe muscle injury. In a subsequent study, patients whose need for physical therapy was not met (as assessed by a physical therapist) were statistically less likely to improve in all selected domains of physical impairment and functional limitation when compared with those patients whose physical therapy needs were met.[22] These 2 studies taken in aggregate seem to show the benefit of physical therapy in severe lower extremity trauma, and suggest that orthopedic surgeons may need to be more aggressive in assisting patients to receive physical therapy.

In conclusion, the LEAP study offers a wide variety of preinjury, injury, treatment, and outcome variables to examine lower extremity injuries. Although treatment was in no way randomized, these articles collectively give enhanced insight into the factors that drive measurable outcomes. Surgeons treating these patients are now more capable of properly counseling the patient and understanding prognostic factors, but perhaps are no better prepared to alter the outcome.

Dr Hansen's quest for a score that will predict which limbs should be salvaged and which should be amputated remains unfulfilled. Ironically, a patient's degree of "self-efficacy" (ie, how well they believe that they can handle change and maximize their future potential) may be the single greatest determining factor studied, and something completely out of the surgeon's control. In the realm of evidence-based medicine, the LEAP studies provided a wealth of data, but still failed to completely determine the treatment at the onset of severe lower extremity trauma.

REFERENCES

1. Hansen ST. The type-IIIC tibial fracture. Salvage or amputation. J Bone Joint Surg Am 1987; 69(6):799–800.

2. Johansen K, Daines M, Howey T, et al. Objective criteria accurately predict amputation following lower extremity trauma. J Trauma 1990;30(5): 568–72 [discussion: 572–3].

3. MacKenzie EJ, Bosse MJ, Kellam JF, et al. Characterization of patients with high-energy lower extremity trauma. J Orthop Trauma 2000;14(7): 455–66.

4. Mackenzie EJ, Bosse M. Factors influencing outcome following limb-threatening lower limb trauma: lessons learned from the Lower Extremity Assessment Project (LEAP). J Am Acad Orthop Surg 2006;14(10 Spec No.):S205–10.

5. Bosse MJ, MacKenzie EJ, Kellam JF, et al. An analysis of outcomes of reconstruction or amputation after leg-threatening injuries. N Engl J Med 2002; 347(24):1924–31.

6. Mackenzie EJ, Bosse MJ, Castillo RC, et al. Functional outcomes following trauma-related lower-extremity amputation. J Bone Joint Surg Am 2004; 86(8):1636–45.

7. Bosse MJ, MacKenzie EJ, Kellam JF, et al. A prospective evaluation of the clinical utility of the lower-extremity injury-severity scores. J Bone Joint Surg Am 2001;83(1):3–14.

8. Bosse M, McCarthy ML, Jones AL, et al. The insensate foot following severe lower extremity trauma: an indication for amputation? J Bone Joint Surg Am 2005;87(12):2601–8.

9. Ly T, Travison T, Castillo R, et al. Ability of lower-extremity injury severity scores to predict functional outcome after limb salvage. J Bone Joint Surg Am 2008;90(8):1738–43.

10. Webb L, Bosse M, Castillo R, et al. Analysis of surgeon-controlled variables in the treatment of limb-threatening type-III open tibial diaphyseal fractures. J Bone Joint Surg Am 2007;89(5):923–8.

11. Castillo R, Bosse M, Mackenzie E, et al. Impact of smoking on fracture healing and risk of complications in limb-threatening open tibia fractures. J Orthop Trauma 2005;19(3):151–7.

12. Pollak AN, McCarthy ML, Burgess AR. Short-term wound complications after application of flaps for coverage of traumatic soft-tissue defects about the tibia. The Lower Extremity Assessment Project (LEAP) Study Group. J Bone Joint Surg Am 2000; 82(12):1681–91.

13. Harris AM, Althausen PL, Kellam J, et al. Complications following limb-threatening lower extremity trauma. J Orthop Trauma 2009;23(1):1–6.

14. O'toole R, Castillo R, Pollak A, et al. Determinants of patient satisfaction after severe lower extremity injuries. J Bone Joint Surg Am 2008;90(6):1206–11.

15. McCarthy ML, Mackenzie E, Edwin D, et al. Psychological distress associated with severe lower-limb injury. J Bone Joint Surg Am 2003; 85(9):1689–97.

16. Patterson B, Agel J, Swiontkowski M, et al. Knee dislocations with vascular injury: outcomes in the Lower Extremity Assessment Project (LEAP) Study. J Trauma 2007;63(4):855–8.

17. Mackenzie EJ, Castillo RC, Jones AS, et al. Health-care costs associated with amputation or reconstruction of a limb-threatening injury. J Bone Joint Surg Am 2007;89(8):1685–92.

18. Mackenzie EJ, Bosse MJ, Pollak AN, et al. Early predictors of long-term work disability after major limb trauma. J Trauma 2006;61(3):688–94.

19. Mackenzie E. Long-term persistence of disability following severe lower-limb trauma. Results of a seven-year follow-up. J Bone Joint Surg Am 2005;87(8):1801–9.

20. Castillo R, Mackenzie E, Wegener ST, et al. Prevalence of chronic pain seven years following limb threatening lower extremity trauma. Pain 2006;124(3):321–9.

21. Castillo R, Mackenzie E, Webb L, et al. Use and perceived need of physical therapy following severe lower-extremity trauma. Arch Phys Med Rehabil 2005;86(9):1722–8.

22. Castillo R, Mackenzie E, Archer KR, et al. Evidence of beneficial effect of physical therapy after lower-extremity trauma. Arch Phys Med Rehabil 2008; 89(10):1873–9.

A Critical Appraisal of the SPRINT Trial

David L. Helfet, MD[a,b,*], Michael Suk, MD, JD, MPH[c,d],
Beate Hanson, MD, PhD[e,f]

KEYWORDS

- Tibial shaft fracture • Intramedullary nails
- Reamed • Unreamed • Randomized controlled trial
- Critical appraisal

Tibial fractures are the most common long-bone fractures, and they are prone to complications such as infections, delayed unions, and nonunions.[1–5] Orthopedic surgeons manage tibial shaft fractures using intramedullary nail fixation, plate fixation, external fixation, and casting or functional bracing.[6–14] A recent consensus among orthopedic surgeons has promoted the use of intramedullary nails in the treatment of tibial shaft fractures.[15–17] Whether the reamed or the unreamed nailing is the optimal treatment remains controversial.[16–19] Unreamed intramedullary nailing may preserve the endosteal blood supply, possibly improve fracture healing, and decrease the risk of infection, whereas the larger reamed intramedullary nails may increase fracture stability.[20–31]

Several small, prospective, randomized controlled trials have compared the effects of reamed intramedullary nailing with those of unreamed intramedullary nailing of lower extremity fractures.[32–36] Recent meta-analyses of these trials have found large reductions in the risk of nonunion or failure of the fracture to heal.[15,16,19,37] The methodological limitations of these trials have left the evidence for either approach inconclusive.[38]

The purpose of this article is to provide an overview and critique of the methodology used by the investigators of the Study to Prospectively evaluate Reamed Intramedullary Nails in Tibial fractures (SPRINT).[38,39]

OVERVIEW OF THE METHODOLOGY USED IN THE SPRINT TRIAL

The SPRINT trial was a multicenter, blinded randomized controlled trial that included 1319 patients with tibial shaft fractures.[39] Twenty-nine centers from the United States, Canada, and the Netherlands participated in the SPRINT trial. The inclusion criteria were men or women who were skeletally mature and had sustained a closed or open fracture of the tibial shaft (Tscherne Type 0–3, Gustilo Type I–IIIB) that was amenable to operative fixation with an intramedullary nail. The exclusion criteria were patients with fractures that were not amenable to intramedullary nailing techniques, those with pathologic fractures, and those who were unlikely to adhere to the follow-up process. Informed consent was obtained from eligible patients who were then randomized to either reamed or unreamed groups using an automated central randomization system. The blinded Outcomes Adjudication Committee adjudicated the eligibility of any randomized patient who did not receive an intramedullary nail. All patients were observed for 1 year.

No funding was received for the preparation of this manuscript.

[a] Weill Cornell Medical College, New York, NY, USA
[b] Orthopaedic Trauma Service, Hospital for Special Surgery, 535 East 70th Street, New York, NY 10021, USA
[c] University of Florida Health Science Center, Jacksonville, FL, USA
[d] Division of Orthopaedic Trauma Surgery, University of Florida—Shands Jacksonville, 655 West 8th Street, ACC Building, 2nd Floor/Ortho, Jacksonville, FL 32209, USA
[e] Department of Health Services, University of Washington, Seattle, USA
[f] AO Foundation, Stettbachstrasse 6, 8600 Duebendorf, Switzerland
* Corresponding author. Orthopaedic Trauma Service, Hospital for Special Surgery, 535 East 70th Street, New York, NY 10021.
E-mail address: helfetd@hss.edu

Orthop Clin N Am 41 (2010) 241–247
doi:10.1016/j.ocl.2009.12.008

Surgical techniques were standardized for the reamed and the unreamed procedures. The study required interlocking of all nails, proximally and distally, and the use of at least 1 proximal locking screw and 1 distal locking screw for all patients. Participating centers standardized key aspects of pre- and postoperative care for closed and open fractures.

The primary outcome was originally defined as a composite outcome that included bone grafting, implant exchange or removal because of a broken nail or deep infection, and debridement of bone and soft tissue because of deep infection. Ineligible events included reoperations planned at the time of the initial surgery and reoperations to promote healing at the site of fractures with a gap of greater than or equal to 1 cm after the initial intramedullary nail fixation. The first interim analysis was conducted when 332 patients were enrolled, and the SPRINT investigators found that the event rate was substantially lower (13%) than that anticipated on the basis of their review of previous studies (32%). In response, they adapted an expanded primary composite outcome that included dynamization of the fracture (ie, interlocking screw removal to allow fracture-site compression with weight bearing); removal of locking screws because of hardware breakage or loosening; autodynamization (spontaneous screw breakage leading to dynamization at the fracture site before healing); fasciotomy; and drainage of hematomas.

Reoperation rates were assessed before hospital discharge and at the time of clinical follow-up visits (2 weeks after discharge and at 6 weeks, 3 months, 6 months, 9 months, and 12 months after surgery). The Adjudication Committee comprised of 5 orthopedic traumatologists, a clinical trialist, and the study statistician, blinded to allocation, adjudicated all potential outcomes to determine if they could be classified as a study event. Disagreements were resolved through discussion and consensus, and all decisions made by the committee were final. At the time of trial closeout, a site audit was conducted to identify any missed potential events.

THE RESULTS OF THE SPRINT TRIAL

Of the 1319 patients randomized into the SPRINT trial, 1226 patients (93%) completed 1 year of follow-up and are included in the analyses.[38] Of these, 622 patients were randomized to the reamed intramedullary nail treatment group and 604 patients to the unreamed group. The patients were predominantly male and involved in motor vehicle–related accidents. Approximately one-third of the patients had sustained an open fracture. The reamed and unreamed treatment groups were similar with respect to key prognostic variables and aspects of operative procedure and perioperative management.

A primary outcome event (relative risk, 0.90; 95% confidence interval, 0.71–1.15; $P = .40$) was experienced by 105 patients (16.9%) in the reamed nailing group and by 114 patients (18.9%) in the unreamed group. Reoperations to promote fracture healing were performed on 106 patients, and 57 of 1226 (4.6%) patients underwent implant exchange or a bone grafting procedure because of nonunion. Of the 106 patients, 48 (45%, including 23 in the reamed nailing group and 25 in the unreamed nailing group; $P = .97$) had a reoperation within 6 months of the original operation. The treatment effect differed across subgroups only between closed and open fractures (test for interaction, $P = .01$).

A total of 113 patients with a closed tibial shaft fracture (13.7%; 95% confidence interval, 12%–16%) underwent a reoperation. Of the patients with closed fractures, 45 of 416 (11%) in the reamed nailing group and 68 of 410 (17%) in the unreamed nailing group experienced a primary event (relative risk, 0.67; 95% confidence interval, 0.47–0.96; $P = .03$). This difference was largely because of differential rates of dynamization, particularly autodynamization.

Of the patients with open tibial shaft fractures, 106 (26.5%; 95% confidence interval, 22%–31%) underwent a reoperation or autodynamization within the first year. In the patients with open fractures, 60 of 206 (29%) in the reamed nailing group and 46 of 194 (24%) in the unreamed nailing group experienced a primary event (relative risk, 1.27; 95% confidence interval, 0.91–1.78; $P = .16$).

The SPRINT investigators concluded that the trial demonstrates a possible benefit for reamed intramedullary nailing in patients with closed fractures. They found no difference between the reoperation rates of reamed and unreamed intramedullary nailing techniques in patients with open fractures. These investigators also reported that delaying reoperations for nonunion for at least 6 months after intramedullary nailing may substantially decrease the need for a reoperation.

CRITICAL APPRAISAL OF THE SPRINT TRIAL METHODOLOGY

This section discusses the validity of the SPRINT trial using the principles outlined in the Users' Guide to the Medical and Surgical Literature.[40,41] The following questions will be applied to the methodology used by the SPRINT investigators: (1) Are the results of the study valid? (2) What are the results? and (3) How can one apply these results to patient care?

Validity

Validity is best assessed as the product of a well-thought-out study design and adherence to principles of randomization, blinding, and patient follow-up.

Q: Were patients randomized?

A: Yes. In the SPRINT trial, patients were randomized to receive either a reamed or an unreamed intramedullary nail, helping to balance known and unknown prognostic factors.[38,39] Factors such as a patient's age, underlying severity of the injury, presence of comorbidities such as diabetes, or health-related habits such as smoking can influence the outcomes of a planned treatment.[40,41] If these factors are influential in selecting the course of treatment for a patient, the outcomes of that treatment will either be underestimated or be overestimated.[40] Because known prognostic factors often influence surgeons' recommendations and patients' treatment decisions, observational studies may yield misleading results.[40] If these factors (both known and unknown) prove unbalanced between a trial's treatment groups, the study's outcome will be biased. The power of randomization is that treatment and control groups are more likely to be balanced with respect to both known and unknown determinants of outcome.[40,42]

Q: Was randomization concealed?

A: Yes. If those making the decision about patient eligibility are aware of the arm of the study to which the patient will be allocated, they may systematically enroll sicker or less sick patients to either of the two treatment groups.[40–42] This may yield a biased result.[40,41] Use of date of birth, odd and even chart numbers, or date of injury, commonly referred to as quasi-randomization methods, results in randomization that is not concealed as the investigator can predict which treatment option the patient will receive.[42] Remote Internet or telephone randomization guarantees concealed randomization.[41,42] Sealed, opaque envelopes that are tamperproof also result in concealed randomization, although remote randomization is more secure.[41]

SPRINT investigators randomized eligible patients by accessing a 24-hour toll-free remote telephone randomization system.[39] This system ensured concealment as it was impossible to predict the patient's treatment group. Randomization was further stratified by the clinical center and the severity of soft tissue injury (open, closed, or both open and closed) in randomly permuted blocks of 2 and 4.[39] The patients and the investigators were unaware of the block sizes, thus further ensuring concealment.[39]

Q: Were all patients analyzed in the groups to which they were randomized?

A: Yes. Under the *intention to treat* principle, all patients were analyzed in the treatment groups to which they were randomized, regardless of the actual treatment received, their eligibility, and whether they followed the study protocol.[41] Excluding patients from analysis in their randomization group for any reason (eg, too sick for surgery) may skew results in favor of a better clinical outcome. Adherence to the *intention to treat* principle preserves the power of randomization by maintaining that important known and unknown prognostic factors are likely to be equally distributed across treatment groups.[42,43] The SPRINT investigators used the *intention to treat* principle.[38,39]

Q: Were patients in the 2 treatment groups similar with respect to known prognostic factors?

A: Yes. In the ideal clinical investigation, differences between the treatment groups are kept at a minimum with regard to known prognostic variables through the process of randomization. Sometimes in trials with small sample sizes and sometimes by chance, randomization fails to result in balanced treatment groups.[40,41]

Large differences in prognostic variables between the 2 treatment groups may compromise the study's validity. Where known prognostic variables have a strong relationship to study outcomes, differences between treatment groups can confound the interpretation of the treatment being studied.[40]

The SPRINT investigators presented multiple prognostic factors by treatment group (eg, age, sex, type of fracture[38]). They reported that the treatment groups were similar with respect to key prognostic variables, making adjustment for any prognostic factors in their analyses unnecessary.[38]

Q: Were patients blinded?

A: Yes. In the SPRINT trial, the patients were blinded to their treatment allocation (reamed vs unreamed intramedullary nailing).[38,39] Patients who believe that one treatment method is more efficacious than the other may feel and perform better than those who do not receive it.[40] Measures such as blinding need to be implemented to ensure that patient reporting is free of influence.[40] These problems can be avoided by ensuring that patients are unaware of the treatment they receive,[40–42] referred to as blinding or masking.[41]

Q: Were treating clinicians blinded?

A: No. Although blinding helps to eliminate the possibility of biased results from differences in patient care,[40] it is particularly challenging to achieve it in randomized controlled trials evaluating different surgical techniques, including the SPRINT trial. This was exacerbated by the preexisting belief among most SPRINT investigators that reamed intramedullary nailing was clinically superior to unreamed intramedullary nailing of tibia fractures.[44] Recognizing that this bias could lead to differences in the threshold for reoperation,[44] a rule was instituted to prevent additional procedures for the treatment of delayed union during the first 6 months after surgery.[38,39] Although adherence to this rule was only 55%, the number of early reoperations was virtually identical in the reamed and unreamed nailing groups.[38] Therefore, this strategy proved to be effective, and study bias was most likely not introduced by a lack of blinding of the attending orthopedic surgeon.

Q: Were outcome assessors blinded?

A: Yes. Unblinded study personnel may influence the results they are measuring or recording through different interpretations of findings or by offering differential encouragement during performance tests.[40] These study personnel can almost always be blinded to the treatment allocation, even if the patient and the treating surgeon cannot.[41] In addition, investigators can have a blinded Adjudication Committee review clinical data to determine whether a patient experienced a study event.[41]

In the SPRINT trial, the blinded Adjudication Committee reviewed all relevant medical records and radiographs to determine if each reported reoperation met the criteria for being a study event.[38,39] An initial concern was whether the size of the nail would be sufficient to unmask the allocation of treatment because the nails used for unreamed fixation are smaller in diameter.[39] To resolve this concern and to keep the committee blinded, the digital radiograph was photo edited to include only the fracture site.[39] Finally, the data analysts were blinded in addition to the Writing Committee who interpreted the results of the trial to prevent bias.[39,45]

Q: Was follow-up complete?

A: Yes. Ideally, investigators would like to know the status of each patient randomized at the conclusion of the trial.[40,42] But, not all patients return for follow-up and consequently are termed "lost to follow-up."[41] These patients may disappear because they suffer adverse outcomes, such as death, or because they are doing well and do not return to be assessed.[40] The greater the number of patients who are lost to follow-up, the more a study's validity is potentially compromised.[41]

Previous randomized controlled trials in orthopedic surgery have typically reported a loss to follow-up rate of 10%, although figures of up to 30% have been reported.[39] The SPRINT investigators implemented numerous strategies to help ensure follow-up, including excluding individuals who were unlikely to keep appointments, obtaining accurate patient contact information and 3 alternate contacts at the time of randomization, organizing the follow-up appointments to coincide with normal surgical fracture clinic visits, and conducting telephone interviews with patients who could not attend the clinic.[39,46]

As a result, 93% of the patients randomized could be observed.[38] However, even a low rate of loss to follow-up may potentially threaten a study's validity. The extent of that compromise remains a matter of judgment and depends on how likely it is that patients lost to follow-up in 1 treatment arm did poorly, whereas patients lost to follow-up in the other treatment arm did well. The SPRINT investigators indicate that the characteristics of the patients who were lost to follow-up were similar to those of the patients who were observed for 1 year.[38] Given both this and their low rate of loss to follow-up, the validity of the SPRINT trial results does not seem to be threatened.

What are the Results?

Q: How large was the treatment effect?

A: Investigators conducting randomized clinical trials carefully monitor how often patients experience adverse events or outcomes.[40,41] These can often be reported as the proportion of patients who experience such an event. The effect of a treatment may also be expressed as a relative risk, which is defined as the ratio of the risk of an event among an exposed population to the risk among the unexposed.[43] The SPRINT investigators appropriately reported their primary composite outcome (reoperation) using relative risks.[38]

Q: How precise was the estimate of the treatment effect?

A: The true risk reduction of a treatment can never be known.[40] The best estimate of it is the point estimate that results from high-quality randomized controlled trials.[40,41] A point estimate is a single value that is calculated from observations of the sample used to estimate a population value or parameter.[40] The point estimate, although close, is unlikely to be precisely correct.[40] The calculation of confidence intervals indicates the range in which the true effect likely lies.[41] A confidence interval is a range of 2 values in which it is probable that the true value lies for the entire population of patients from which the study patients were selected.[43] A 95% confidence interval defines the range that includes the true relative risk reduction 95% of the time.[40] The SPRINT investigators appropriately reported 95% confidence intervals around each relative risk.[38]

How Can One Apply the Results to Patient Care?

Q: Were the study patients similar to my patient?

A: Sufficient details on both patient and fracture characteristics[38,39] to allow readers to make a comparison with the patients they see in their own clinical practice were presented.[40] Inclusion and exclusion criteria were also clearly listed.

Q: Were all clinically important outcomes considered?

A: It is necessary to critically assess whether a trial reports all the important outcomes.[40] In the SPRINT trial, the primary composite outcome was measured postoperatively at 12 months and included bone grafting, implant exchange, and dynamization in patients with a fracture gap of less than 1 cm.[38] Infection and fasciotomy were considered as part of the composite outcome, irrespective of the postoperative gap.[38] Adverse events were also reported, including death, deep venous thrombosis, pulmonary embolus, and sepsis.[38] Patient-reported measures, such as health-related quality of life, were assessed but not presented in the primary manuscript.[47]

Q: Are the likely treatment benefits worth the potential harm and costs?

A: Yes. It is also necessary to ascertain if the probable treatment benefits are worth the additional effort and costs.[40] The SPRINT trial results have important implications for clinical practice as a possible benefit for reamed intramedullary nailing in patients with closed fractures was demonstrated.[38] No difference was found between reamed or unreamed approaches in patients with open fractures.[38] In addition, the trial's results suggest that the level of reoperations may be reduced by allowing increased time for these fractures to heal.[38]

SUMMARY

Orthopedic trauma research has recently undergone a paradigm shift from single-center randomized controlled trials to larger multicenter ones,[48–50] allowing more patients to be recruited in a much quicker time frame and increasing the generalizability of the results. Conducting a multicenter randomized controlled trial is complex and time consuming; so rigorous methodology must be followed.

The strengths of the successful SPRINT trial included a large sample size; multiple participating surgeons and centers; strategies to reduce bias, which included centralized randomization to ensure concealment; blinding of patients, data analysts, and the individuals interpreting the results of the analysis; independent, blinded adjudication of patient eligibility and outcomes; and a proscription of reoperation for nonunion before 6 months.[38,39] Given the high methodological rigor of this multicenter initiative, the results of the SPRINT trial should not only change clinical practice but also set a benchmark for the conduct of future trials in orthopedic surgery. In conclusion, the SPRINT trial provides an example of a well-conducted multicenter randomized controlled trial.

REFERENCES

1. Russell TA. Fractures of the tibial diaphysis. In: Levine AM, editor. Orthopaedic knowledge update trauma. Rosemont (IL): American Academy of Orthopaedic Surgeons; 1996. p. 171–9.

2. Turen CH, Burgess AR, Vanco B. Skeletal stabilization of tibial fractures associated with acute compartment syndrome. Clin Orthop Relat Res 1995;315:163–9.

3. Watson JT, Anders M, Moed B. Management strategies for bone loss in tibial fractures. Clin Orthop 1995;315:138–53.

4. Burgess AR, Poka A, Brumback RJ, et al. Pedestrian tibial injuries. J Trauma 1987;27:596–601.

5. Blick SS, Brumback RJ, Poka A, et al. Compartment syndrome in open tibial fractures. J Bone Joint Surg Am 1986;68(9):1348–53.

6. Helfet DL, Haas NP, Schatzker J, et al. Philosophy and principles of fracture —its evolution and evaluation. J Bone Joint Surg Am 2003;85(6):1156–60.

7. Anglen JO, Blue JM. A comparison of reamed and unreamed nailing of the tibia. J Trauma 1995;39: 351–5.

8. Boynton MD, Curcin A, Marino AR. Intramedullary treatment of open tibial fractures: a comparative study. Orthop Trans 1992;16:662.

9. Court-Brown CM, McQueen MM, Quaba AA, et al. Locked intramedullary nailing of open tibial fractures. J Bone Joint Surg Br 1991;73(6):959–64.

10. Clifford RP, Beauchamp CG, Kellam JF, et al. Plate fixation of open fractures of the tibia. J Bone Joint Surg Br 1988;70(4):644–8.

11. McGraw JM, Lim EV. Treatment of open tibial shaft fractures: external fixation and secondary intramedullary nailing. J Bone Joint Surg Am 1988;70(6):900–11.

12. Den Outer AJ, Meeuwis JD, Hermans JZA. Conservative versus operative treatment of displaced non-comminuted tibial shaft fractures: a retrospective comparative study. Clin Orthop Relat Res 1990; 252:231–7.

13. Digby JM, Holloway GM, Webb JK. A study of function after tibial cast bracing. Injury 1983;14:432–9.

14. Hooper GJ, Keddell RG, Penny ID. Conservative management or closed nailing for tibial shaft fractures: a randomised prospective trial. J Bone Joint Surg Br 1991;73(1):83–5.

15. Littenberg B, Weinstein LP, McCarren M, et al. Closed fractures of the tibial shaft: a meta-analysis of three methods of treatment. J Bone Joint Surg Br 1998;80:174–83.

16. Bhandari M, Guyatt GH, Tong D, et al. Reamed versus nonreamed intramedullary nailing of lower extremity long bone fractures: a systematic overview and meta-analysis. J Orthop Trauma 2000;14:2–9.

17. Bhandari M, Guyatt GH, Swiontkowski MF, et al. Treatment of open fractures of the shaft of the tibia. J Bone Joint Surg Br 2001;83:62–8.

18. Bhandari M, Guyatt GH, Tornetta P 3rd, et al. Current practice in the intramedullary nailing of tibial shaft fractures: an international survey. J Trauma 2002; 53(4):725–32.

19. Forster MC, Bruce AS, Aster AS. Should the tibia be reamed when nailing? Injury 2005;36:439–44.

20. Rhinelander FW. Tibial blood supply in relation to fracture healing. Clin Orthop Relat Res 1974;105: 34–81.

21. Rhinelander FW. The vascular response of bone to internal fixation. In: Browner BD, Edwards CC, editors. The science and practice of intramedullary nailing. Philadelphia: Lea and Febiger; 1987. p. 25–9.

22. Olerud S, Strömberg L. Intramedullary reaming and nailing: its early effects on cortical bone vascularization. Orthopedics 1986;9:1204–8.

23. Klein MP, Rahn BA, Frigg R, et al. Reaming versus non-reaming in medullary nailing: interference with cortical circulation of the canine tibia. Arch Orthop Trauma Surg 1990;109:314–6.

24. Hupel TM, Aksenov SA, Schemitsch EH. Cortical bone blood flow in loose and tight fitting locked intramedullary nailing: a canine segmental tibia fracture model. J Orthop Trauma 1998;12:127–35.

25. Schemitsch EH, Turchin DC, Kowalski MJ, et al. Quantitative assessment of bone injury and repair after reamed and unreamed locked intramedullary nailing. J Trauma 1998;45:250–5.

26. Schemitsch EH, Kowalski MJ, Swiontkowski MF. Soft-tissue blood flow following reamed versus unreamed locked intramedullary nailing: a fractured sheep tibial model. Ann Plast Surg 1996;36:70–5.

27. Utvåg SE, Grundnes O, Reikerås O. Effects of degrees of reaming on healing of segmental fractures in rats. J Orthop Trauma 1998;12:192–9.

28. Grundnes O, Utvåg SE, Reikerås O. Restoration of bone flow following fracture and reaming in rat femora. Acta Orthop Scand 1994;65:185–90.

29. Fairbank AC, Thomas D, Cunningham B, et al. Stability of reamed and unreamed intramedullary tibial nails: a biomechanical study. Injury 1995;26:483–5.

30. Whittle AP, Wester W, Russell TA. Fatigue failure in small diameter tibial nails. Clin Orthop Relat Res 1995;315:119–28.

31. Bhandari M, Schemitsch EH. Bone formation following intramedullary femoral reaming is decreased by indomethacin and antibodies to insulin-like growth factors. J Orthop Trauma 2002; 16:717–22.

32. Keating JF, O'Brien PJ, Blachut PA, et al. Locking intramedullary nailing with and without reaming for open fractures of the tibial shaft: a prospective, randomized study. J Bone Joint Surg Am 1997;79: 334–41.

33. Finkemeier CG, Schmidt AH, Kyle RF, et al. A prospective, randomized study of intramedullary nails inserted with and without reaming for the treatment of open and closed fractures of the tibial shaft. J Orthop Trauma 2000;14:187–93.

34. Blachut PA, O'Brien PJ, Meek RN, et al. Interlocking intramedullary nailing with and without reaming for the treatment of closed fractures of the tibial shaft. A prospective, randomized study. J Bone Joint Surg Am 1997;79(5):640–6.

35. Court-Brown CM, Will E, Christie J, et al. Reamed or unreamed nailing for closed tibial fractures. A prospective study of Tscherne C1 fractures. J Bone Joint Surg Br 1996;78:580–3.

36. Tornetta P III, Tiburzi D. The treatment of femoral shaft fractures using intramedullary interlocked nails with and without intramedullary reaming: a preliminary report. J Orthop Trauma 1997;11: 89–92.

37. Coles CP, Gross M. Closed tibial shaft fractures: management and treatment complications. A review of the prospective literature. Can J Surg 2000;43: 256–62.

38. SPRINT Investigators, Bhandari M, Guyatt G, et al. Randomized trial of reamed and unreamed intramedullary nailing of tibial shaft fractures. J Bone Joint Surg Am 2008;90(12):2567–78.

39. SPRINT Investigators, Bhandari M, Guyatt G, et al. Study to prospectively evaluate reamed intramedullary nails in patients with tibial fractures (S.P.R.I.N.T.): study rationale and design. BMC Musculoskelet Disord 2008;9:91.

40. Guyatt G, Rennie D, Meade MO, et al. Users' guides to the medical literature: a manual for evidence-based clinical practice. 2nd edition. USA: McGraw Hill Medical; 2008. American Medical Association.

41. Bhandari M, Guyatt GH, Swiontkowski MF. User's guide to the orthopaedic literature: how to use an

article about a surgical therapy. J Bone Joint Surg Am 2001;83(6):916–26.

42. Hanson B. Designing, conducting and reporting clinical research: a step by step approach. Injury 2006;37:583–94.

43. Bhandari M, Tornetta P 3rd, Guyatt GH. Glossary of evidence-based orthopaedic terminology. Clin Orthop Relat Res 2003;413:158–63.

44. Devereaux PJ, Bhandari M, Clarke M, et al. Need for expertise based randomised controlled trials. BMJ 2005;330:88.

45. Boutron I, Estellat C, Guittet L, et al. Methods of blinding in reports of randomized controlled trials assessing pharmacologic treatments: a systematic review. PLoS Med 2006;3(10):e425.

46. Sprague S, Leece P, Bhandari M, et al. S.P.R.I.N.T. Investigators. Limiting loss to follow-up in a multicenter randomized trial in orthopedic surgery. Control Clin Trials 2003;24:719–25.

47. S.P.R.I.N.T. Investigators, Tornetta P. A Randomized Trial of Reamed versus Non-Reamed Intramedullary Nail Insertion on Functional Outcome in Patients with Fractures of the Tibia. Orthopaedic Trauma Association (OTA) 23rd Annual Meeting. Boston, MA, October 19, 2007.

48. Wright JG, Gebhardt MC. Multicenter clinical trials in orthopaedics: time for musculoskeletal specialty societies to take action. J Bone Joint Surg Am 2005;87:214–7.

49. Trippel SB, Bosse MJ, Heck DA, et al. Symposium. How to participate in orthopaedic randomized clinical trials. J Bone Joint Surg Am 2007;89:1856–64.

50. Bhandari M, Sprague S, Schemitsch EH, International Hip Fracture Research Collaborative. Resolving controversies in hip fracture care: the need for large collaborative trials in hip fractures. J Orthop Trauma 2009;23(6):479–84.

Graft Selection for Anterior Cruciate Ligament Reconstruction: A Level I Systematic Review Comparing Failure Rates and Functional Outcomes

Keith R. Reinhardt, MD[a,b,*], Iftach Hetsroni, MD[c], Robert G. Marx, MD, FRCSC[b]

KEYWORDS

- Anterior cruciate ligament
- Bone-patellar tendon-bone composites
- Combined semitendinosus and gracilis hamstring tendons
- Revision

Tear of the anterior cruciate ligament (ACL) is the most common ligamentous injury of the knee. Reconstructing this ligament is often required to restore functional stability of the knee.[1,2] Despite the popularity of the procedure, the preferred graft remains controversial. Ideally, the graft should have similar characteristics as the native ACL. Regardless of graft type, the biologic and mechanical properties of the graft material should provide a favorable setting for early biologic incorporation, be amenable to secure fixation, and limit potential morbidity related to donor site.

Many graft options are available for ACL reconstruction, including different autograft and allograft tissues. Autografts include bone-patellar tendon-bone composites (PT), combined semitendinosus and gracilis hamstring tendons (HT), and quadriceps tendon. Allograft options include the same types of tendons harvested from donors, in addition to Achilles and tibialis tendons. Tissue-engineered anterior cruciate grafts are not yet available for clinical use, but may become a feasible alternative in the future.

For the past few decades, PT autograft has been the gold standard for ACL reconstruction. Reasons for this include the strength of the tissue, relative ease of harvest, and bone-to-bone healing with secure fixation. More recently, HT autografts have joined PT in surgeons' popularity.[3] The recent trend toward increased use of HT resulted from concerns with use of PT relating to a potential negative effect on the knee extensor mechanism and donor site morbidity, including anterior knee pain and risk for patella fracture.[4] Nevertheless, despite their increasing popularity, HT grafts also have potential limitations, including slower soft-tissue graft-tunnel healing compared with bone-to-bone healing with PT grafts, potential for tunnel

[a] 310 East 71st Street, Apartment 2L, New York, NY 10021, USA
[b] Department of Orthopedic Surgery, Hospital for Special Surgery, Weill Medical College of Cornell University, 535 East 70th Street, New York, NY 10021, USA
[c] Orthopedic Department, Meir General Hospital, Tsharnichovski Street 59, Kfar Saba 44281, Israel
* Corresponding author.
E-mail address: reinhardtk@hss.edu

Orthop Clin N Am 41 (2010) 249–262
doi:10.1016/j.ocl.2009.12.009

orthopedic.theclinics.com

Table 1
Details of studies

Study	Year of Publication	Mean Age (Years) (Range) PT	HT	Sample Size (N) (% Follow-up)	Mean Follow-up (Months)	Number of HT Strands	PT Tibia	PT Femur	HT Tibia	HT Femur
Aglietti et al[10]	1994	NA		60 (95)	28	4	IfSc	ScW	ScW	ScW
Aglietti et al[11]	2004	25 (16–39)	25 (15–39)	120 (100)	24	4	IfSc	S	ScW	Sc
Anderson et al[12]	2001	23.6 (14–44)	21 (14–40)	68 (97)	35	2	St	IfSc	Su	St
Beynnon et al[13]	2002		29.2 (18–46)	44 (79)	36	2	IfSc	IfSc	St	St
Biau et al[14,c]	2007	NA		1263 (NA)	NA	2, 3, 4 or 5	Variable	Variable	Variable	Variable
Ejerhed et al[15]	2003	26 (14–49)	29 (15–59)	66 (93)	24	3 or 4	IfSc	IfSc	IfSc	IfSc
Eriksson et al[16]	2001		25.7	154 (94)	33	4	IfSc	IfSc	Sc	Eb
Feller & Webster[17]	2003	26.3	25.8	57 (88)	36	4	IfSc	Eb	Post	Eb
Grontvedt et al[18,b]	1996		26 (16–48)	92 (92)	24	0	IfSc	IfSc + St	IfSc + St	IfSc + St
Harilainen et al[19]	2006	31		79 (80)	60	4	IfSc	IfSc	ScW	P
Ibrahim et al[20]	2005		22.3 (17–34)	85 (77)	81	4	IfSc	Eb	ScW, P + St	P
Jansson et al[21]	2003	NA		89 (90)	24	4	IfSc	IfSc	ScW	P
Laxdal et al[22]	2005	28 (16–52)	25 (12–41)	118 (88)	26	3 or 4	IfSc	IfSc	IfSc	IfSc
Liden et al[23]	2007	28 (14–49)	29 (15–59)	68 (96)	86	3 or 4	IfSc	IfSc	IfSc	IfSc
Maletis et al[24]	2007	27.2 (15–42)	27.7 (14–48)	96 (97)	24	4	IfSc	IfSc	2 IfSc	IfSc

Study	Year	Age	Age	N (%)	N		PW	PW	PW	PW	PW
Marder et al[25]	1991	21.6 (16–35)	23.8 (17–41)	72 (90)	29	4	IfSc	IfSc	IfSc	IfSc	IfSc
Matsumoto et al[26]	2006	23.7	24.4	72 (90)	87	5	St	St	St	St	IfSc
Moyen et al[27,b]	1992	24	24	64 (64)	36	0	St	St	St	St	St
Muren et al[28,b]	2003	25 (20–33)	25 (19–44)	40 (100)	84	0	Su	Post + Su	Su	Su	ScW
O'Neill[29]	1996		27 (14–56)	125 (98)	42	2	IfSc or St	IfSc	IfSc	St	St
O'Neill[30]	2001	NA	NA	225 (95)	102	2	IfSc or St	IfSc	IfSc	St	St
Sajovic et al[31]	2006	27 (16–46)	24 (14–42)	54 (84)	60	4	IfSc	IfSc	IfSc	IfSc	IfSc
Shaieb et al[32]	2002	32 (14–48)	30 (14–53)	70 (85)	33	4	IfSc	IfSc	IfSc	IfSc	IfSc
Sun et al[33,a]	2009	29.7 (16–59)	30.1 (20–63)	65 (96)	31	0	IfSc	IfSc	IfSc	IfSc	IfSc
Sun et al[34,a]	2009	31.7 (20–54)	32.8 (19–65)	156 (93)	67	0	IfSc	IfSc	IfSc	IfSc	IfSc
Taylor et al[35]	2009	21.7 (18–37)	22.1 (17–44)	53 (83)	36	4	IfSc + ScW	IfSc + Eb	IfSc + ScW	IfSc + Eb	IfSc + Eb
Webster et al[36]	2001	26	27	61 (94)	24	4	IfSc	Eb	Post + Su	Eb	Eb
Zafagnini et al[37]	2006	30.5 (22–47)	29 (15–49)	75 (100)	60	2 or 4	IfSc	IfSc	IfSc ± St	IfSc ± St	Eb ± St

Abbreviations: Eb, endobutton; IfSc, interference screw; NA, not available; P, plate; PW, post + washer; Sc, screw; St, staples; Su, sutures; ScW, screw and washer.

a PT autograft compared with PT allograft.
b Comparison made with PT with KLAD.
c Meta-analysis.

Table 2
Quality assessment of study methodology

Study	Randomization Method	Selection Bias	Performance Bias	Detection Bias	Attrition Bias
Aglietti et al[10]	Alternating sequence	+	−	+	−
Aglietti et al[11]	Alternating sequence	+	−	−	−
Anderson et al[12]	Computer-generated	−	−	+	−
Beynnon et al[13]	Random numbers table	−	−	+	+
Biau et al[14,c]	Variable	+	−	−	−
Ejerhed et al[15]	Sealed envelopes	+	−	−	−
Eriksson et al[16]	NA	+	−	−	−
Feller&Webster[17]	Computer-generated	−	−	−	−
Grontvedt et al[18,b]	Sealed envelopes	+	−	+	−
Harilainen et al[19]	Even/odd birth year	+	−	+	+
Ibrahim et al[20]	Even/odd birth year	+	−	+	+
Jansson et al[21]	Even/odd birth year	+	−	+	+
Laxdal et al[22]	Sealed envelopes	+	−	−	+
Liden et al[23]	Sealed envelopes	+	−	−	+
Maletis et al[24]	Computer-generated	+	−	−	−
Marder et al[25]	Alternating sequence	+	−	+	−
Matsumoto et al[26]	Even/odd birth year	+	−	+	−
Moyen et al[27,b]	Drawing of lots	−	−	+	+
Muren et al[28,b]	Random sealed envelopes	−	−	+	−
O'Neill[29]	Birth month allocation	+	−	+	−
O'Neill[30]	Birth month allocation	+	−	+	−
Sajovic et al[31]	Even/odd registration number	−	−	+	−
Shaieb et al[32]	Even/odd birth year	+	−	+	−
Sun et al[33,a]	Computer-generated	−	−	+	−
Sun et al[34,a]	Computer-generated	−	−	+	−
Taylor et al[35]	Random sealed envelopes	−	−	+	−
Webster et al[36]	Computer-generated	−	−	+	−
Zafagnini et al[37]	Alternating sequence	+	−	+	−

Abbreviations: +, bias present in the study; NA, not available.
[a] PT autograft compared with PT allograft.
[b] Comparison made with PT with KLAD.

widening and graft laxity, and functional hamstring weakness resulting from graft harvesting.[5,6]

There are several randomized controlled trials (RCTs) in the literature comparing the two most popular graft choices, PT and HT, either used as autografts or allografts. Many of the systematic reviews and meta-analyses in the literature that investigate graft choice for ACL reconstruction are biased by their inclusion of inadequately randomized trials that are not true level I studies.[7–9] Also, functional outcomes, rather than graft failure, tend to be the focus of these reviews. The authors believe, however, that graft failure represents a critically important outcome measure in ACL reconstruction, which has not been given enough attention in previous systematic reviews and meta-analyses. The purpose of this systematic review is to assess whether one of the popular grafts (PT and HT) is preferable for reconstructing the ACL. For this objective the authors selected only true level I studies that compared these graft choices in functional clinical outcomes, failure rates, and other objective parameters following reconstruction of the ACL.

METHODS

A systematic literature review was performed using the following data sources: MEDLINE with OVID and PubMed (basic search, related articles, clinical queries search), EMBASE, and the Cochrane Central Register of Controlled Trials for relevant articles in the English language. Bibliographies of the identified articles on this topic were also reviewed. In addition, a manual search of recent pertinent hard copy journals from the previous 6 months was undertaken to identify journal articles that may not yet have been included in electronic databases.

Initial inclusion criteria included prospective RCTs, meta-analyses of RCTs, studies comparing PT and HT, either autografts or allografts, for ACL reconstruction, minimum of 2-year follow-up after the reconstruction for RCTs but not for meta-analyses of RCTs, no restrictions on date of publication or publication status. Following this initial search the inclusion criteria were further refined to include, in addition to the above criteria, only properly randomized trials comparing 2-strand HT or 4-strand HT with PT autografts. The criteria for proper randomization were strict to avoid any potential selection bias. Proper randomization techniques included random numbers table, computer-generated randomization, and randomly ordered sealed envelopes. Trials using even and odd birth years/months, patient registration numbers, or another alternating sequence of

allocation were excluded because of inadequate randomization and the associated potential bias.

All studies identified in the initial search were screened for duplications by entering them into a computer-based reference management system. All eligible articles were then screened first by title and abstract, followed by an in-depth review of the methodology and outcomes. The results of this search are shown in **Tables 1** and **2**, which include studies with proper randomization techniques and those that were quasi-randomized. Following this, the authors limited the review further to studies with appropriate randomization only, as described earlier. A standardized data extraction form was modified and used to retrieve data from each article on study design, population, interventions, and outcomes.[38] Outcomes of particular interest included return to preinjury level of activity, graft failure rate, donor site morbidity, laxity measurements, knee range of motion, isokinetic muscle strength, and standardized knee outcomes scores. The authors defined graft failure rate as either revision ACL reconstruction or a 2-plus positive pivot shift test. KT-1000 measurements were not included as a criterion for failure because of variability in testing and because the pivot shift test is associated with function, whereas the KT-1000 is not.[39]

The quality of the studies, including internal and external validity, was appraised using the items contained in the CONSORT Statement: Revised Recommendations for Improving the Quality of Reports of Parallel-Group Randomized Trials.[38] Furthermore, each study was assessed for the 4 main biases affecting method quality: selection bias, performance bias, detection bias, and attrition bias.

RESULTS
General Description of Studies

Twenty-eight studies published between 1991 and 2009 (27 prospective RCTs and 1 meta-analysis of RCTs) met the initial inclusion criteria (see **Table 1**). The data for each study were collected using a worksheet developed by the authors. The basic details of the studies are shown in **Table 1**, including sample sizes, length of follow-up, and methods of fixation of the grafts. Of the 28 studies, 23 prospectively compared PT autografts with 2-, 3-, 4-, or 5-strand semitendinosus and gracilis (HT) composite autografts (including 1 meta-analysis of studies comparing PT autografts with HT autografts of varying sizes).[10–17,19–26,29–32,35–37] Three studies compared PT autografts with PT autografts augmented by the Kennedy ligament augmentation device (KLAD),[18,27,28] and two studies compared PT autografts with PT fresh-frozen allografts, which were γ-irradiated in 1 study[33] and nonirradiated in the other.[34]

Study Design Appraisal

The presence of the 4 main biases affecting study quality, and the treatment allocation methods used in each of the studies, are shown in **Table 2**. Each of the studies in the initial stage of this review allocated patients during the same period in a prospective random fashion, either by computer-generated random models or via quasi-randomized allocation methods (ie, birth date, alternating sequence, sealed envelopes that were not randomly ordered).

Detection bias can be minimized by blinding patients and investigators at follow-up evaluations. No patient in any study was blinded to the type of graft they received, but several independent follow-up evaluations were performed by blinded investigators, and the outcomes of the treatment groups in each study were assessed in identical fashion, thereby minimizing detection bias (see **Table 2**).

Attrition bias pertains to loss of patients from treatment groups after allocation, by either late exclusion or lost to follow-up. As shown in **Table 2**, several studies excluded patients after treatment allocation, but 1 study[27] had more than 30% lost to follow-up, which has been reported as the threshold for acceptable follow-up, with less than 20% being preferable.[40] Another study had 23% lost to follow-up.[20] Attrition bias was also prevalent in another study,[21] and in its subsequent study with longer follow-up,[19] in which data from 4 graft failures (all in the HT group) were excluded in the final analysis. This finding may represent a systematic exclusion of data that could potentially overestimate the favorable results in the HT group. Graft failures were similarly excluded from final data analysis in another study.[23] As graft failure rate is a critical outcome following ACL reconstruction, methodology that excludes failures from the final analysis limits the value of the conclusions reached in these studies.

To improve the validity of our conclusions, our analysis of functional clinical outcomes, failure rates, and other objective parameters was limited to RCTs that had proper randomization (ie, computer-based, random numbers table, random sealed envelopes), and 80% follow-up at a minimum of 2 years follow-up. Also, as discussed earlier, trials comparing PT with HT were required to use HT composites of 2- or 4-strand quadrupled grafts only. Studies not meeting these strict criteria were excluded from all subsequent analyses, leaving 6 of 28 studies. Of these, 4 studies compared PT autografts with 4-strand HT autografts,[17,24,35,36] and two studies compared PT autografts with 2-strand HT autografts.[12,13] These 6 studies served as the basis for our analyses and subsequent conclusions. One study had a follow-up rate of 79% and we elected to include it.

OUTCOMES
Graft Failure Rate

In the 6 studies that met the inclusion criteria, the authors evaluated graft failure rates and included all patients with a final follow-up pivot shift test of 2+ or greater or patients who required revision ACL surgery (**Table 3**). The results of the graft failure analysis are shown in **Table 3**. In the two

Table 3
ACL graft failure (defined as 2+ positive pivot shift or ACL revision reconstruction)

Study	Sample Size (N)			Graft Failure (Number of Patients) (%)	
	Total	PT	HT	PT	HT
Anderson et al[12,b]	68	35	33	7 (20)	8 (24.2)
Beynnon et al[13,b]	44	22	22	0	6 (27.3)
Feller & Webster[17]	57	26	31	1 (3.8)	5 (16.1)
Maletis et al[24]	96	46	50	0	2 (4.0)
Taylor et al[35]	53	24	29	3 (12.5)	5 (17.2)
Webster et al[36]	61	28	33	NR	NR
Totals	379	181	198	11 (7.2)[a]	26 (15.8)[a]

Abbreviation: NR, not reported.
[a] Patients from Webster et al[36] were not included in total ACL graft failure calculations because this was not reported in their study. Inclusion criteria: properly randomized controlled trials comparing PT autograft with 2-strand or 4-strand HT autograft, and minimum 2 years' follow-up with 80% complete follow-up (1 study had 79% follow-up).
[b] Comparison between PT and 2-strand HT.

studies that compared PT with 2-strand HT auto-grafts,[12,13] 7 graft failures were seen in 57 PT reconstructions (12.3%), whereas 14 graft failures occurred in 55 HT reconstructions (25.5%). In the 4 studies that used 4-strand HT as the comparison graft, 4 PT graft failures were seen in 96 recon-structions (4.2%), and 12 failures occurred in 110 4-strand HT reconstructions (10.9%). The graft failure rate was significantly higher in the Beynnon study that compared PT with 2-strand HT (P = .024). Overall the graft failure rate for the 6 studies was 11 failures out of 153 reconstructions in the PT groups (7.2%) and 26 failures out of 165 recon-structions in the HT groups (15.8%) (P = .02).

Knee Range of Motion

All 6 studies, in some fashion, reported on range of motion deficits at final follow-up **(Table 4)**. Neither of the two studies comparing PT with 2-strand HT found a significant difference in knee range of motion.[12,13] Two of the 4 studies that compared PT with 4-strand HT found significantly higher extension deficits in the PT groups (see **Table 4**).[17,36] Neither of the remaining two studies reported significant differences in knee range of motion.

Patellofemoral Pain

In this review, 5 of the 6 included studies reported on donor site morbidity, specifically patellofemoral pain **(Table 5)**. Of the 2 studies comparing PT with 2-strand HT, one study reported on patellofemoral crepitus and found no significant difference,[12] and the other looked at the incidence of anterior knee pain and again found no significant difference.[13] Three studies comparing PT with 4-strand HT used patient reports of pain with kneeling, or diffi-culty or inability to walk on their knees, as a surro-gate for patellofemoral pain. Of those 3 studies, 1 found a significantly higher incidence of pain with kneeling and knee-walking in the PT group (P<.01).[17] That same study also presented subjec-tive patient reports of anterior knee pain, and found significantly more subjective anterior knee pain in the PT group (P<.05). Of the 4 studies that found no significant differences statistically in knee pain outcomes, 3 of them reported higher absolute pain scores in the PT groups, and one study reported higher absolute pain ratings in the HT group (see **Table 5**).

Activity Level and Functional Assessments

As shown in **Table 6**, studies used various measures of patient activity for preinjury and follow-up assessments **(Tables 6** and **7)**. Neither study that used 2-strand HT as the comparison group found

significant differences in final follow-up activity levels compared with PT (see **Table 6**). Of the 4 studies comparing PT with 4-strand HT, 2 studies found significant differences in activity level at final follow-up, one of which found a significantly higher percentage of patients in the PT groups returning to their preinjury level of activity compared with the HT groups.[24] However, in that particular study the preinjury Tegner activity level was found to be signif-icantly lower in the PT group (P = .03), which theo-retically could have made it easier for PT patients to return to their preinjury activity level because it was lower to start with. **Table 7** contains the data on standardized functional outcome assessments for each of the studies.

Anterior Knee Laxity

All the studies in this review included instru-mented-laxity testing as an objective outcome measure **(Table 8)**. As seen in **Table 8**, both studies comparing PT with 2-strand HT grafts re-ported significantly more laxity in the 2-strand HT grafts at final follow-up.[12,13] One of 4 studies comparing PT with 4-strand HT found higher laxity in the HT group (P<.05).[17] All studies, except one,[35] reporting side-to-side differences of a 3-mm threshold reported higher absolute values of anterior laxity in the HT groups compared with the PT groups.

Isokinetic Muscle Strength

Five of the 6 studies reported on isokinetic muscle strength testing of the quadriceps and hamstrings muscles at final follow-up **(Table 9)**. As shown in **Table 9**, the only significant difference in muscle strength found between PT and 2-strand HT grafts was a greater peak hamstring muscle torque deficit at 240 degrees/s in the 2-strand HT group (P = .04).[13] Also, two of the 3 studies comparing PT with 4-strand HT showed significantly more hamstring weakness in the HT autograft groups.[17,24] Only 1 study found significantly weak-er quadriceps in the PT autograft group (P = .04).[24]

DISCUSSION

Over the past two decades, the most commonly asked question in ACL surgery has been "what is the best graft option?" From this systematic review, since 1991 27 prospective RCTs and 1 meta-analysis of RCTs meeting the authors' initial inclusion criteria have been conducted looking for the answer to this question. These studies for the most part compared PT autografts with HT auto-grafts; however, 3 of them compared PT auto-grafts with PT autografts plus KLAD,[18,27,28] and 2 studies used PT allografts[33,34] (1 γ-irradiated,

Table 4
Knee range of motion deficits at final follow-up

Study	Extension Deficits (Number of Patients) (%) PT		HT		Flexion Deficits (Number of Patients) (%) PT		HT		Comments
	3–5°	≥5°	3–5°	≥5°	3–5°	≥5°	3–5°	≥5°	
Anderson et al[12,a]	3 (9)	0	1 (2)	7 (10)	0	1 (3)	0	10 (15)	NS
Beynnon et al[13,a]	—	—	—	—	—	—	—	—	Deficits reported as means (NS)
Feller & Webster[17]	—	—	—	—	—	—	—	—	Extension deficit means: PT 2.7, HT 1.2 (P<.05)
Maletis et al[24]	—	—	—	—	—	—	—	—	Deficits reported as means (NS)
Taylor et al[35]	—	—	—	—	—	—	—	—	Deficits reported as means (NS)
Webster et al[36]	6 (26)	4 (17)	4 (13)	1 (3)	—	—	—	—	P<.05

Abbreviations: —, unclear from presentation of data within the study, not reported, or categorized differently by study; NS, no significant difference.
[a] Comparison between PT and 2-strand HT.

Table 5
Patellofemoral pain at latest follow-up

Study	Patellofemoral Crepitus (Number of Patients) (%) PT	HT	P	Pain with Kneeling or Knee-Walking (Number of Patients) (%) PT	HT	P	Anterior Knee Pain (Number of Patients) (%) PT	HT	P
Anderson et al[12,a]	9 (26)	14 (21)	NS						
Beynnon et al[13,a]							7 (32)	5 (23)	NS
Feller & Webster[17]				17 (67)	8 (26)	<0.01	11 (43)	10 (33)	<0.05
Maletis et al[24]				9 (20)	3 (6)	NS			
Taylor et al[35]				2 (9.5)	5 (20.8)	NS			
Webster et al[36]	NR	NR		NR	NR		NR	NR	

Abbreviations: NR, not reported; NS, no significant difference; P, P value.
[a] Comparison between PT and 2-strand HT.

Table 6
Preinjury and latest follow-up activity levels after ACL reconstruction

Study	Preinjury Activity Level				Latest Follow-up Activity Level			
	Scale	PT	HT	P	Scale	PT	HT	P
Anderson et al[12,a,b]	NR	NR	NR		IKDC level I	83%	81%	NS
Beynnon et al[13,a,b]	NR	NR	NR		Tegner/IKDC level I	4/59%	4/45%	NS
Feller & Webster[17]	Cincinnati activity score	91.6 (8)[b]	87.3 (13)[b]	NS	Cincinnati level I	27%	36%	NS
Maletis et al[24]	Tegner	6.8	7.2	0.03	Return to preinjury Tegner	51%	26%	0.01
Taylor et al[35]	NR	NR	NR		Tegner	6.8	5.3	0.04
Webster et al[36]	NR	NR	NR		IKDC level I or II	61.3%	60.9%	NS

Abbreviations: IKDC, International Knee Documentation Committee; NR, preinjury activity level not reported; NS, no significant difference; P, P value.
[a] Comparison between PT and 2-strand HT.
[b] Number in parentheses denotes standard deviation.

Table 7
Functional assessments at latest follow-up

Study	IKDC Score (% Normal/Nearly Normal)			Lysholm Score (Mean)			Cincinnati Score (Mean) (SD)		
	PT	HT	P	PT	HT	P	PT	HT	P
Anderson et al[12,a]	97	73	0.02						
Beynnon et al[13,a]	NA	NA		NA	NA		NA	NA	
Feller & Webster[17]	71	93	NS				92.7 (9.0)	93.7 (8.2)	NS
Maletis et al[24]				97	98	NS			
Taylor et al[35]	86	78	NS	90.4	90.3	NS			
Webster et al[36]	61	61	NS						

Abbreviations: IKDC, International Knee Documentation Committee; NA, not applicable to study; NS, no significant difference; P, P value.
[a] Comparison between PT and 2-strand HT.

Table 8
Objective knee stability testing at final follow-up

Study	Instrument	Force	≥3 mm Side-to-Side Difference			Mean Laxity (mm) (SD)		
			PT (%)	HT (%)	P	PT	HT	P
Anderson et al[12,a]	KT-1000 arthrometer	Manual maximum	29	48	NS	2.1 (2.0)	3.1 (2.3)	<0.05
Beynnon et al[13,a]	KT-1000 arthrometer	133 N	23	55	0.004	1.1	4.4	0.001
Feller & Webster[17]	KT-1000 arthrometer	134 N	5	15	NS	0.5 (1.5)	1.6 (1.3)	<0.05
Maletis et al[24]	KT-1000 arthrometer	Manual maximum				2.3	2.8	NS
Taylor et al[35]	KT-2000 arthrometer	134 N	50	36.4	NS			
Webster et al[36]	KT-1000 arthrometer	30 pounds	7.1	9.1	NS	1.1	1.7	NS

Abbreviations: N, newtons; NS, no significant difference; P, P value.
[a] Comparison between PT and 2-strand HT.

one nonirradiated fresh-frozen) as the comparison group. The criteria by which all of these studies have attempted to judge the superiority of one graft to another include the rate of graft failure, knee range of motion, donor site morbidity, quadriceps/hamstring muscle strength, anterior knee laxity, return to preinjury activity level, and standardized functional knee outcome scores.

In the authors' opinion, the two most important issues for patients who have undergone ACL reconstruction are knee stability (in the relative short-term) and the development of osteoarthritis (in the long-term). The latter requires decades of follow-up and it is not yet possible to determine from the literature whether one graft source has a higher risk than another for the development of degenerative changes. On a more basic level, ACL reconstruction is performed to provide a stable knee for the patient. If this is not achieved, then the operation has not accomplished the main

Table 9
Isokinetic strength of the quadriceps and hamstrings (reported as % of contralateral uninvolved knee)

Study	Instrument	Speed (Degrees/s)	Knee Extension (Quadriceps) (%)			Knee Flexion (Hamstrings) (%)		
			PT	HT	P	PT	HT	P
Anderson et al[12,a]	Cybex II	60	86	96	NS	96	96	NS
		180	91	99	NS	100	96	NS
Beynnon et al[13,a]	Cybex	60	94.7	88.1	NS	99.4	95.5	NS
		180	95.9	92.1	NS	95.8	90.9	NS
		240	96.6	93.5	NS	100.3	89.3	0.04
Feller & Webster[17]	Cybex II	60	77.3	88.9	NS	98.3	92.3	<0.05
		240	85.2	91	NS	99.4	105.5	NS
Maletis et al[24]	Dynamometer (Biodex)	60	85	92	0.04	99	91	NS
		180	93	96	NS	102	90	0.0001
		300	94	96	NS	96	93	NS
Taylor et al[35]	Dynamometer (Biodex)	60	87.9	96.9	NS	83.2	97.5	NS
		300	91.6	94.3	NS	95.9	100.3	NS
Webster et al[36]	NR	NR	NR	NR		NR	NR	

Abbreviations: NR, not reported; NS, no significant difference; P, P value.
[a] Comparison between PT and 2-strand HT.

goal. Stability can be challenging to define and is affected by many factors, not the least of which is patient activity level. To clarify this definition, we selected two end points that we felt clearly indicated that stability was not achieved: documentation of a positive pivot shift test and revision ACL reconstruction. Although it is possible that a patient may have an unstable knee without a detectable pivot shift on examination, the authors believed that if either of these two outcomes was documented, then the procedure could clearly be considered a failure.

Most of the randomized clinical trials comparing graft sources have significant potential biases that could affect the conclusions. In an attempt to eliminate this potential problem, the authors further refined the analysis, limiting it only to trials that compared PT with either 2-strand or 4-strand HT autografts, trials that used appropriate methods of randomization, and that had a minimum of 2 years' follow-up with 80% follow-up. These criteria eliminated 22 of 28 studies, leaving 6 trials. Using these 6 studies with these criteria for failure, PT autografts had 11 failures of 153 cases (7.2%) and HT autografts had 26 failures of 165 cases (15.8%). This difference in failure rate using only the best evidence available is important clinical information that has not been previously reported. Although fixation and other techniques used in the studies vary, this difference in graft failure rate is statistically significant and clinically meaningful.

Other outcomes are discussed in detail in the results section. Overall, there is a trend toward increased donor site morbidity in PT autografts compared with HT autografts. The authors believe that this potential increase in morbidity is better tolerated by younger, more active patients who also have a higher risk of graft failure.[41] Therefore the authors favor PT autografts for younger patients who tend to have fewer problems caused by donor site morbidity and who also have a higher risk of re-tearing their graft.

Aside from clinical outcomes, there are biologic and biomechanical aspects of the various grafts that are useful to explore. For ideal reconstruction and postoperative rehabilitation planning, ACL graft selection should take into consideration the following factors: graft tissue mechanical properties compared with native ACL properties, the time frame for solid biologic graft incorporation, the mechanical stability of the initial fixation technique and device used, and the effect of the sterilization method on the quality of the tissue when using allograft.

Biomechanical testing in cadaveric knees of the native human femur-ACL-tibia complex in anatomic orientation to maximize stiffness and load to failure has shown that younger specimens (22–35 years) demonstrate the highest values of linear stiffness (242 N/mm) and ultimate load to failure (2160 N), whereas older specimens (60–97 years) demonstrate the lowest values of linear stiffness (180 N/mm) and ultimate load to failure (658 N).[42] Comparing mechanical characteristics of different ACL grafts is challenging because of study methodology differences in graft size, age, orientation of specimen, and methods of testing and fixation devices. Nevertheless, tensile properties and load to failure of several graft tissues provide some helpful information for graft selection.

Bone-patellar composites, investigated in vitro, have demonstrated mechanical properties comparable to the native ACL. Nonetheless, some investigators have suggested a possible correlation between mechanical characteristics of the graft and donor age.[43,44] Load to failure of 10-mm patellar tendon-bone composites was around 2900 N when donor tissue was from a young group (average age 28 years), and was comparable to thicker grafts (14 mm) obtained from an older population.[43,44] On the other hand, other investigators did not find a correlation between mechanical characteristics of patellar tendon grafts and age between 18 and 55 years.[45]

For human hamstring quadruple grafts, the composite was stiffer (776 N/mm) and had higher loads to failure (4090 N) compared with previously described 10-mm patellar tendon grafts, supporting its use from a mechanical standpoint as an ACL graft tissue.[46] From a surgical technical standpoint all 4 strands of the graft must be under equal tension for the composite to have its optimum biomechanical properties. Other soft-tissue grafts such as doubled tibialis anterior, doubled tibialis posterior, and doubled peroneus longus have also been measured mechanically, and have demonstrated load to failure of around 3000 N and stiffness of around 300 N/mm.[47]

Although less popular for ACL reconstruction, quadriceps tendon has also been tested mechanically and was found to have comparable mechanical properties to patellar tendon tissue (1.36 times load to failure compared with similar width patellar tendon graft, which was not statistically significant), and thus is appropriate also for ACL reconstruction.[48]

With regard to allograft tissue, the sterilization process may affect the mechanical characteristics of the tissue and therefore should also be thought of when selecting a graft. This process is necessary to decrease viral disease transmission and bacterial infection rate, but it may also adversely affect the quality of the tissue. Several techniques have been used for this purpose. Although ethylene oxide sterilization does not alter directly the mechanical properties of the graft, it has been shown to cause clinical failure because of persistent synovitis, and therefore is less favorable.[49,50] Another sterilization technique involves applying γ-irradiation. High-dose irradiation (3 Mrad or more) is unacceptable as it severely affects mechanical properties of the tissue. Irradiation (2–2.5 Mrad) has also been shown in several studies to cause unacceptable inferior clinical outcomes and high failure rates.[51,52]

The use of allograft tissue has increased significantly in the past decade because of increased availability and the elimination of donor site morbidity. However, Carey and colleagues[53] have recently demonstrated that there are limited data from randomized trials. Most case series include a smaller number of young patients (ie, less than 30 years of age) and there have been early reports of unacceptably high failure rates in young patients.[54,55] Furthermore, procurement, storage, sterilization, and processing vary widely within the industry and the authors encourage all surgeons to be familiar with the methods and standards of the tissue bank they use. The authors currently use allograft tissue for certain revision and multiligament cases, and primary ACL reconstruction in patients who are typically more than 40 years of age, not active in highly aggressive cutting and pivoting sports, and who wish to minimize donor site morbidity related to graft harvest.

SUMMARY

When only high-quality randomized clinical trials are evaluated, the risk of graft failure is significantly higher with hamstring tendon reconstruction compared with patellar tendon autograft. This difference has been discussed but not demonstrated previously because of bias in study design and inadequate power. The authors believe this finding is particularly important when selecting a graft for higher-risk patients who are sufficiently skeletally mature for patellar tendon autograft ACL reconstruction.

REFERENCES

1. Daniel DM, Stone ML, Dobson BE, et al. Fate of the ACL-injured patient. A prospective outcome study. Am J Sports Med 1994;22(5):632–44.

2. Fithian DC, Paxton LW, Goltz DH. Fate of the anterior cruciate ligament-injured knee. Orthop Clin North Am 2002;33(4):621–36, v.

3. McRae S, Chahal J, Leiter J, et al. A survey study of members of the Canadian Orthopaedic Association regarding the natural history and treatment of anterior cruciate ligament injury. AOSSM Annual Meeting. Keystone, Colorado, July 97–12, 2009.

4. Biau DJ, Tournoux C, Katsahian S, et al. Bone-patellar tendon-bone autografts versus hamstring autografts for reconstruction of anterior cruciate ligament: meta-analysis. BMJ 2006;332(7548): 995–1001.

5. Hollis R, West H, Greis P, et al. Autologous bone effects on femoral tunnel widening in hamstring anterior cruciate ligament reconstruction. J Knee Surg 2009;22(2):114–9.

6. Bizzini M, Gorelick M, Munzinger U, et al. Joint laxity and isokinetic thigh muscle strength characteristics after anterior cruciate ligament reconstruction: bone patellar tendon bone versus quadrupled hamstring autografts. Clin J Sport Med 2006;16(1):4–9.

7. Herrington L, Wrapson C, Matthews M, et al. Anterior cruciate ligament reconstruction, hamstring versus bone-patella tendon-bone grafts: a systematic literature review of outcome from surgery. Knee 2005; 12(1):41–50.

8. Spindler KP, Kuhn JE, Freedman KB, et al. Anterior cruciate ligament reconstruction autograft choice: bone-tendon-bone versus hamstring: does it really matter? A systematic review. Am J Sports Med 2004;32(8):1986–95.

9. Poolman RW, Abouali JA, Conter HJ, et al. Overlapping systematic reviews of anterior cruciate ligament reconstruction comparing hamstring autograft with bone-patellar tendon-bone autograft: why are they different? J Bone Joint Surg Am 2007;89(7):1542–52.

10. Aglietti P, Buzzi R, Zaccherotti G, et al. Patellar tendon versus doubled semitendinosus and gracilis tendons for anterior cruciate ligament reconstruction. Am J Sports Med 1994;22(2):211–7 [discussion: 217–8].

11. Aglietti P, Giron F, Buzzi R, et al. Anterior cruciate ligament reconstruction: bone-patellar tendon-bone compared with double semitendinosus and gracilis tendon grafts. A prospective, randomized clinical trial. J Bone Joint Surg Am 2004;86(10):2143–55.

12. Anderson AF, Snyder RB, Lipscomb AB Jr. Anterior cruciate ligament reconstruction. A prospective randomized study of three surgical methods. Am J Sports Med 2001;29(3):272–9.

13. Beynnon BD, Johnson RJ, Fleming BC, et al. Anterior cruciate ligament replacement: comparison of bone-patellar tendon-bone grafts with two-strand hamstring grafts. A prospective, randomized study. J Bone Joint Surg Am 2002;84(9):1503–13.

14. Biau DJ, Tournoux C, Katsahian S, et al. ACL reconstruction: a meta-analysis of functional scores. Clin Orthop Relat Res 2007;458:180–7.

15. Ejerhed L, Kartus J, Sernert N, et al. Patellar tendon or semitendinosus tendon autografts for anterior cruciate ligament reconstruction? A prospective

randomized study with a two-year follow-up. Am J Sports Med 2003;31(1):19–25.

16. Eriksson K, Anderberg P, Hamberg P, et al. A comparison of quadruple semitendinosus and patellar tendon grafts in reconstruction of the anterior cruciate ligament. J Bone Joint Surg Br 2001; 83(3):348–54.

17. Feller JA, Webster KE. A randomized comparison of patellar tendon and hamstring tendon anterior cruciate ligament reconstruction. Am J Sports Med 2003;31(4):564–73.

18. Grontvedt T, Engebretsen L, Bredland T. Arthroscopic reconstruction of the anterior cruciate ligament using bone-patellar tendon-bone grafts with and without augmentation. A prospective randomised study. J Bone Joint Surg Br 1996;78(5):817–22.

19. Harilainen A, Linko E, Sandelin J. Randomized prospective study of ACL reconstruction with interference screw fixation in patellar tendon autografts versus femoral metal plate suspension and tibial post fixation in hamstring tendon autografts: 5-year clinical and radiological follow-up results. Knee Surg Sports Traumatol Arthrosc 2006;14(6): 517–28.

20. Ibrahim SA, Al-Kussary IM, Al-Misfer AR, et al. Clinical evaluation of arthroscopically assisted anterior cruciate ligament reconstruction: patellar tendon versus gracilis and semitendinosus autograft. Arthroscopy 2005;21(4):412–7.

21. Jansson KA, Linko E, Sandelin J, et al. A prospective randomized study of patellar versus hamstring tendon autografts for anterior cruciate ligament reconstruction. Am J Sports Med 2003;31(1):12–8.

22. Laxdal G, Kartus J, Hansson L, et al. A prospective randomized comparison of bone-patellar tendon-bone and hamstring grafts for anterior cruciate ligament reconstruction. Arthroscopy 2005;21(1): 34–42.

23. Liden M, Ejerhed L, Sernert N, et al. Patellar tendon or semitendinosus tendon autografts for anterior cruciate ligament reconstruction: a prospective, randomized study with a 7-year follow-up. Am J Sports Med 2007;35(5):740–8.

24. Maletis GB, Cameron SL, Tengan JJ, et al. A prospective randomized study of anterior cruciate ligament reconstruction: a comparison of patellar tendon and quadruple-strand semitendinosus/gracilis tendons fixed with bioabsorbable interference screws. Am J Sports Med 2007;35(3):384–94.

25. Marder RA, Raskind JR, Carroll M. Prospective evaluation of arthroscopically assisted anterior cruciate ligament reconstruction. Patellar tendon versus semitendinosus and gracilis tendons. Am J Sports Med 1991;19(5):478–84.

26. Matsumoto A, Yoshiya S, Muratsu H, et al. A comparison of bone-patellar tendon-bone and bone-hamstring tendon-bone autografts for anterior cruciate ligament reconstruction. Am J Sports Med 2006;34(2):213–9.

27. Moyen BJ, Jenny JY, Mandrino AH, et al. Comparison of reconstruction of the anterior cruciate ligament with and without a Kennedy ligament-augmentation device. A randomized, prospective study. J Bone Joint Surg Am 1992; 74(9):1313–9.

28. Muren O, Dahlstedt L, Dalen N. Reconstruction of acute anterior cruciate ligament injuries: a prospective, randomised study of 40 patients with 7-year follow-up. No advantage of synthetic augmentation compared to a traditional patellar tendon graft. Arch Orthop Trauma Surg 2003;123(4):144–7.

29. O'Neill DB. Arthroscopically assisted reconstruction of the anterior cruciate ligament. A prospective randomized analysis of three techniques. J Bone Joint Surg Am 1996;78(6):803–13.

30. O'Neill DB. Arthroscopically assisted reconstruction of the anterior cruciate ligament. A follow-up report. J Bone Joint Surg Am 2001;83(9):1329–32.

31. Sajovic M, Vengust V, Komadina R, et al. A prospective, randomized comparison of semitendinosus and gracilis tendon versus patellar tendon autografts for anterior cruciate ligament reconstruction: five-year follow-up. Am J Sports Med 2006;34(12):1933–40.

32. Shaieb MD, Kan DM, Chang SK, et al. A prospective randomized comparison of patellar tendon versus semitendinosus and gracilis tendon autografts for anterior cruciate ligament reconstruction. Am J Sports Med 2002;30(2):214–20.

33. Sun K, Tian SQ, Zhang JH, et al. ACL reconstruction with BPTB autograft and irradiated fresh frozen allograft. J Zhejiang Univ Sci B 2009;10(4):306–16.

34. Sun K, Tian SQ, Zhang JH, et al. Anterior cruciate ligament reconstruction with bone-patellar tendon-bone autograft versus allograft. Arthroscopy 2009; 25(7):750–9.

35. Taylor DC, DeBerardino TM, Nelson BJ, et al. Patellar tendon versus hamstring tendon autografts for anterior cruciate ligament reconstruction: a randomized controlled trial using similar femoral and tibial fixation methods. Am J Sports Med 2009;37(10):1946–57.

36. Webster KE, Feller JA, Hameister KA. Bone tunnel enlargement following anterior cruciate ligament reconstruction: a randomised comparison of hamstring and patellar tendon grafts with 2-year follow-up. Knee Surg Sports Traumatol Arthrosc 2001;9(2):86–91.

37. Zaffagnini S, Marcacci M, Lo Presti M, et al. Prospective and randomized evaluation of ACL reconstruction with three techniques: a clinical and radiographic evaluation at 5 years follow-up. Knee Surg Sports Traumatol Arthrosc 2006; 14(11):1060–9.

38. Wright RW, Brand RA, Dunn W, et al. How to write a systematic review. Clin Orthop Relat Res 2007; 455:23–9.

39. Kocher MS, Steadman JR, Briggs KK, et al. Relationships between objective assessment of ligament stability and subjective assessment of symptoms and function after anterior cruciate ligament reconstruction. Am J Sports Med 2004;32(3):629–34.

40. Greenhalgh T. How to read a paper: the basics of evidence based medicine. London: BMJ Publishing Group; 2001.

41. Lyman S, Koulouvaris P, Sherman S, et al. Epidemiology of anterior cruciate ligament reconstruction: trends, readmissions, and subsequent knee surgery. J Bone Joint Surg Am 2009;91(10):2321–8.

42. Woo SL, Hollis JM, Adams DJ, et al. Tensile properties of the human femur-anterior cruciate ligament-tibia complex. The effects of specimen age and orientation. Am J Sports Med 1991;19(3):217–25.

43. Noyes FR, Butler DL, Grood ES, et al. Biomechanical analysis of human ligament grafts used in knee-ligament repairs and reconstructions. J Bone Joint Surg Am 1984;66(3):344–52.

44. Cooper DE, Deng XH, Burstein AL, et al. The strength of the central third patellar tendon graft. A biomechanical study. Am J Sports Med 1993;21(6): 818–23 [discussion: 823–4].

45. Flahiff CM, Brooks AT, Hollis JM, et al. Biomechanical analysis of patellar tendon allografts as a function of donor age. Am J Sports Med 1995;23(3): 354–8.

46. Hamner DL, Brown CH Jr, Steiner ME, et al. Hamstring tendon grafts for reconstruction of the anterior cruciate ligament: biomechanical evaluation of the use of multiple strands and tensioning techniques. J Bone Joint Surg Am 1999;81(4):549–57.

47. Pearsall AW 4th, Hollis JM, Russell GV Jr, et al. A biomechanical comparison of three lower extremity tendons for ligamentous reconstruction about the knee. Arthroscopy 2003;19(10):1091–6.

48. Harris NL, Smith DA, Lamoreaux L, et al. Central quadriceps tendon for anterior cruciate ligament reconstruction. Part I: morphometric and biomechanical evaluation. Am J Sports Med 1997;25(1):23–8.

49. Jackson DW, Windler GE, Simon TM. Intraarticular reaction associated with the use of freeze-dried, ethylene oxide-sterilized bone-patellar tendon-bone allografts in the reconstruction of the anterior cruciate ligament. Am J Sports Med 1990;18:1–11.

50. Roberts TS, Drez D Jr, McCarthy W, et al. Anterior cruciate ligament reconstruction using freeze-dried, ethylene oxide-sterilized, bone-patellar tendon-bone allografts. Two year results in thirty-six patients. Am J Sports Med 1991;19(1):35–41.

51. Rappe M, Horodyski M, Meister K, et al. Nonirradiated versus irradiated Achilles allograft: in vivo failure comparison. Am J Sports Med 2007;35(10): 1653–8.

52. Sun K, Tian S, Zhang J, et al. Anterior cruciate ligament reconstruction with BPTB autograft, irradiated versus non-irradiated allograft: a prospective randomized clinical study. Knee Surg Sports Traumatol Arthrosc 2009;17(5):464–74.

53. Carey JL, Dunn WR, Dahm DL, et al. A systematic review of anterior cruciate ligament reconstruction with autograft compared with allograft. J Bone Joint Surg Am 2009;91(9):2242–50.

54. Kaeding CC, Pedroza A, Aros BC, et al. Independent predictors of ACL reconstruction failure from the MOON prospective longitudinal cohort. AOSSM Annual Meeting. Orlando, Florida, July 10–13, 2008.

55. Luber KT, Greene PY, Barrett GR. Allograft anterior cruciate ligament reconstruction in the young, active patient (Tegner activity level and failure rate). AOSSM Annual Meeting. Orlando, Florida, July 10–13, 2008.

Hip Resurfacing Arthroplasty: A Review of the Evidence for Surgical Technique, Outcome, and Complications

Derek F. Amanatullah, MD, PhD, Yeukkei Cheung, MD,
Paul E. Di Cesare, MD*

KEYWORDS

- Hip • Resurfacing • Surface • Replacement
- Arthroplasty • Metal-on-metal • Alternate bearing

Many patients seek hip arthroplasty earlier in life to remain physically active rather than accept the limitations of their hip arthritis. This younger patient demographic will likely require additional hip surgery because the life expectancy of patients in their 40s and 50s will most likely exceed 30 more years.[1] As a result, the lack of established longevity for standard bearing (metal-on-polyethylene) total hip arthroplasty (THA) and the need for future revision of THA in this younger patient population has prompted the use of alternative bearing surfaces and fueled the resurgence of hip resurfacing arthroplasty.

The first hip resurfacing procedures (large metal head articulating with high-molecular-weight polyethylene) performed in the 1970s resulted in an unacceptably high wear rate resulting in failure secondary to osteolysis (ie, aseptic loosening or inflammatory bone resorption).[2–4] Despite this initial failure, efforts have been made to improve surgical technique, instrumentation, and implant design.At present, there are several hip resurfacing implant systems available; however, only the Cormet (Corin, England) and Birmingham hip

resurfacing systems (Smith and Nephew, Memphis, TN, USA) are approved by the Food and Drug Administration for use in the United States.[4]

MODERN IMPLANT DESIGN

Current hip resurfacing implants use a metal-on-metal bearing surface, with implants forged or cast from high-carbon cobalt-chromium-molybdenum alloy. If the femoral and acetabular implants are well-manufactured and well-positioned, large-diameter metal-on-metal bearing surfaces are predicted by lubrication theory to produce very low levels of volumetric wear compared with the metal-on-polyethylene surfaces used in the past.[5–9]

Hybrid fixation (press-fit acetabular and cemented femoral components) is most commonly used. A cementless acetabular cup is typically press fit into the under-reamed acetabulum. The acetabular cup has a surface modification of cobalt-chromium beads or plasma-sprayed titanium with or without hydroxyapatite coating for bone in-growth and fixation.[10,11] The femoral

Disclosures: The authors of this article have received no benefits, funding, or support in conjunction with this report.
Department of Orthopaedic Surgery, University of California Davis Medical Center, 4860 Y Street, Suite 3800, Sacramento, CA 95817, USA
* Corresponding author.
E-mail address: paul.dicesare@ucdmc.ucdavis.edu

Orthop Clin N Am 41 (2010) 263–272
doi:10.1016/j.ocl.2010.01.002

component is traditionally cemented into place on the femoral neck. There are, however, cementless designs being used because of the potential for thermal bone necrosis during the cement curing process, contributing to early implant failure.[12–15]

SURGICAL TECHNIQUE

There is no ideal surgical approach for hip resurfacing arthroplasty.[16–21] There is a balance between the risks of surgical dissection and necessary exposure and visualization. Femoral head oxygen concentration is compromised in both the anterolateral and posterior approaches. However, during the anterolateral approach and not the posterior approach, femoral oxygen concentration recovers after implantation with hip relocation (**Table 1**), suggesting compromise of the ascending branch of the medial circumflex femoral artery during release of the short external

rotators during the posterior approach.[22,23] However, a posterior approach used in surgical dislocation that protects the tendon of the obturator externus and consequently the ascending branch of the medial circumflex femoral artery has no risk of femoral head osteonecrosis (see **Table 1**).[24,25] Retrieval studies demonstrated osteonecrosis of the remaining femoral head in 10 of 14 failed hip resurfacing arthroplasties using the posterior approach; 9 underwent revision for femoral neck fracture, and 1 underwent revision for femoral component loosening.[26]

Preparation of the femoral head by reaming is enough to decrease blood flow to the femoral head by 70% in 9 of 10 hips.[27] This is likely a result of disruption of the nutrient retinacular vessels of the femoral head because 80% of these vessels penetrate bone in the anterosuperior and posterosuperior quadrants of the femoral neck.[28] Valgus positioning during reaming results in notching of

Table 1
Established technical considerations during hip resurfacing arthroplasty and their corresponding highest level of evidence

Technical Considerations	Evidence	Citations
The anterolateral approach preserves the blood supply to the femoral head	Level III, B	22
The extended posterior approach compromises the blood supply to the femoral head	Level IV, B	23,26
An obturator externus tendon sparing posterior approach does not compromise the blood supply to the femoral head	Level IV, B	24,25
Reaming of the femoral head decreases blood supply to the femoral head	Level IV, B	27
Femoral neck notching decreases blood supply to the femoral head and is associated with femoral implant loosening	Level IV, B	29,30
A cement mantle more than 3 mm is associated with femoral implant loosening	Level IV, B	12
Filling of bone cysts greater than 1 cm^3 is associated with femoral implant loosening	Level IV, B	12,62
Lesser trochanteric suction cannula can control femoral temperatures during cementing	Level III, B	13
A varus stem-shaft angle less than 130° correlates with adverse outcome	Level III, B	35
Hip resurfacing arthroplasty cannot dramatically affect limb length or horizontal femoral offset	Level III, B	39,40
Biomechanical reconstruction of the hip is comparable to THA with hip resurfacing arthroplasty if minimal initial deformity is present	Level I, A	41
Acetabular bone loss is similar to that of THA	Level I, A	39,42
Acetabular component abduction angle of greater than 55° can increase wear	Level IV, B	12,15
Femoral bone stock is preserved and may be converted to THA	Level II, B	44,45,48,49

Level of evidence Data from the *Journal of Bone and Joint Surgery* (I–IV) and the *Orthopedic Clinics of North America* (A or B).

the femoral neck and a reduction of blood flow by 50% in 10 of 14 hips by laser Doppler flowmetry (see **Table 1**).[29] Notching is associated with an increase in femoral component loosening, from 6.8% to 28.6%, during radiographic follow-up of 72 hip resurfacing arthroplasties (see **Table 1**).[30] Removal of up to 30% of the anterolateral femoral neck does not alter the load-bearing capacity of the proximal femur, suggesting that there is minimal mechanical weakness attributed to femoral neck notching and that there is a vascular component to femoral neck notching that contributes to loosening as opposed to fracture.[29,31–33]

The heat produced by polymerization of the cement that is used to fix the femoral component may result in thermal bone necrosis.[14] Retrieval studies of 96 failed hip resurfacing arthroplasties demonstrate that femoral implants that failed secondary to femoral loosening had an average cement mantle of 2.9 mm, whereas nonfemoral failures had an average cement mantel of 2.3 mm. In addition, the bone-cement interface of the loose femoral components were thick, fibrous, and associated with bone resorption, and the interface of those isolated for femoral neck fracture were ischemic. Cement-filled bone cysts were more prevalent in hip resurfacing arthroplasties that failed secondary to femoral loosening. Finite element modeling supports the concept that deep cement penetration or filling of a bone cyst larger than 1 cm^3 results in temperatures that are consistent with thermal bone necrosis (see **Table 1**).[12] Another retrieval study that evaluated 55 failed hip resurfacings supports these conclusions.[15] Use of a 3-mm suction cannula inserted into a hole drilled in the lesser trochanter, penetrating 3 cm into the intramedullary canal for femoral preparation and cementing, resulted in a decrease in the maximal femoral temperature from 68°C to 36°C, well below the level required for thermal bone necrosis (see **Table 1**).[13]

The positioning of the femoral component is critical.[34] Evaluation of 94 hip resurfacing arthroplasties showed that a varus stem-shaft angle, less than 133°, correlated with adverse outcomes (see **Table 1**).[35] Finite element analysis supports placement of the femoral implant in a relative valgus position as a result of decreased predicted peak stress levels more similar to those of a normally loaded femur (**Fig. 1**).[36,37] Valgus positioning by 10° increased load to fracture by 28%.[38] However, radiographic studies demonstrate that placement of the femoral component in 5° to 10° of relative valgus position slightly decreases mean femoral offset by 4.5 to 8 mm and results in mean limb length discrepancy of −2.2 to 0.3 mm (see **Table 1**).[39,40] Hence, hip resurfacing arthroplasty can

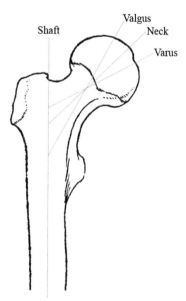

Fig. 1. Depiction of normal femoral neck shaft angle (125° between shaft and neck) as well as varus (greater than 130° between shaft and implant) and valgus (less than 130° between shaft and implant) hip resurfacing arthroplasty positioning. Note that valgus positioning aligns the femoral component with the medial cortical structures. (*From* Freeman MA. Some anatomic and mechanical considerations relevant to the surface replacement of the femoral head. Clin Orthop Relat Res 1978;134:19–24; with permission.)

only minimally alter hip biomechanics to correct deformity. Despite this limitation, a randomized clinical trial of 120 patients comparing THA to hip resurfacing arthroplasty confirmed a mean limb shortening of 1.9 mm and a mean reduction in horizontal offset by 3.3 mm in the hip resurfacing arthroplasty limb of the study (see **Table 1**).[41]

Despite issues with exposure, reaming, and cementing, the modern metal-on-metal hybrid hip resurfacing implants provide the bone stock conservation required for the implant to be viable in a younger patient population (see **Table 1**). Many acetabular components require the removal of less than 5 mm of acetabular bone stock, similar to the amount of acetabular bone stock removed during a THA. A randomized trial of 230 hips demonstrated no difference in the size of the acetabular component in hip resurfacing arthroplasty or THA.[39,42] Positioning of the acetabular component is also important because an abduction angle (ie, lateral opening angle) of greater than 55° has been shown to increase wear in simulation and retrieval studies.[12,15,43]

The conservation of bone stock on the femoral side is intuitive because a hip resurfacing arthroplasty can easily be converted to a THA in the case of complication or need for revision.[44–47] There is no demonstrated loss of bone mineral density secondary to stress shielding during hip resurfacing arthroplasty in comparative studies.[48,49] However, there is a 70% incidence of femoral neck narrowing seen during retrospective review of 163 hip resurfacing arthoplasties.[50] The consequence of this finding is unknown.

MODERN HIP RESURFACING ARTHROPLASTY OUTCOMES

Hip resurfacing arthroplasty has been shown to be equivalent to THA in short- to medium-term retrospective studies (**Table 2**). Comparison of 52 hip resurfacing arthroplasties with 93 cementless THAs after a mean follow-up of 3 years revealed similar revision rates of 3.5% and 4.3%, respectively. In addition, the complication rate and improvements in function, range of motion, and pain were also similar.[51] The 5-year mean follow-up data on age, gender, body mass index, and activity level were also similar between hip resurfacing arthroplasty and hybrid THA, with 6% and 8% revision rates, respectively, and with similarly excellent quality of life and functional scores.[52] The Australian Orthopaedic Association National Joint Replacement Registry supports these findings. Men younger than 65 years with hip resurfacing arthroplasty have a similar revision rate to those with THA. The

revision rate of hip resurfacing arthroplasty is 2% at 5 years.[53] Harris Hip Scores are equivalent at 2 years in retrospective comparison of 337 hip resurfacing arthroplasties and 266 THAs.[54] Gait is also shown to be similar between patients who underwent hip resurfacing arthroplasty and those who underwent THA, with the former group walking at almost a normal speed of 1.26 m/s.[55] A prospective, randomized, controlled trial comparing 48 patients demonstrated no difference in gait speed or postural balance. In fact, both groups had reached normal parameters at 3 months post surgery.[56] There are several unpublished reports and trials showing that range of motion after hip resurfacing arthroplasty is full in all planes of motion, but retrospective data show an almost 20° increase in hip flexion after surgery to greater than 110°.[57,58] A retrospective study supports the concept that early hip resurfacing arthroplasty results in an improved functional outcome (see **Table 2**). Hips with fewer changes secondary to osteoarthritis (ie, bone density, femoral neck shape, hip biomechanics, and focal bone defects) correlated with improved postoperative hip pain, range of motion, and biomechanics and fewer acetabular radiolucencies.[59]

Patient selection remains critical to obtaining excellent results. Two case series support the concept that hip resurfacing arthroplasty in active men younger than 55 years with osteoarthritis can result in satisfactory implant survivorship (see

Table 2
Established patient criteria for optimal hip resurfacing arthroplasty outcomes and expected outcomes after hip resurfacing arthroplasty and their corresponding highest level of evidence

Patient Selection and Outcome	Evidence	Citations
Hip resurfacing arthroplasty survivorship at 3 and 5 years is equivalent to THA	Level II, B	51–53
0.02% revision rate in men younger than 55 years with osteoarthritis	Level IV, B	60,61
3% revision rate if SARI[a] ≤3; 11% revision rate if SARI>3	Level IV, B	62
Patients return to a high level of function, including sports, after hip resurfacing arthroplasty	Level I, A	60,62,63,66
Gait speed and postural balance are similar to THA and normal at 3 months postsurgery	Level I, A	55,56
Hip flexion increases by 20° after hip resurfacing arthroplasty	Level IV, B	57,58
Early intervention favors a good functional outcome	Level II, B	59
Patients with osteonecrosis of the femoral head have an increased revision rate of 7%	Level II, B	67,68

[a] SARI is calculated by summing assigned numbers for specific risks: 1 for previous surgery, 2 if less than 82 kg, 1 for high activity, and 2 for femoral cysts greater than 1 cm.
  Data from Beaule PE, Dorey FJ, LeDuff M, et al. Risk factors affecting outcome of metal-on-metal surface arthroplasty of the hip. Clin Orthop Relat Res 2004;418:87–93. Level of evidence from the *Journal of Bone and Joint Surgery* (I–IV) and the *Orthopedic Clinics of North America* (A or B).

Table 2). About 446 hip resurfacing arthroplasties performed on young men with osteoarthritis showed a 0.02% revision rate with a mean follow-up of 3.3 years despite the high activity level of the men in the series. Thirty percent of the men were involved in jobs that they considered heavy or moderately heavy, and 87% of men participated in leisure-time sporting activity, and none were instructed to change their level of activity after the procedure.[60] A smaller case series on a similar patient demographic demonstrates a 99% implant survivorship for aseptic cases after a slightly longer mean follow-up of 5 years.[61] Two other series evaluating 230 hip resurfacing arthroplasties at 3- and 5-years mean follow-up demonstrate 99.1% survivorship at each interval.[57,58] A case series (using less strict selection criteria) of 400 hip resurfacing arthroplasties (average age of patients, 48 years; 73% male; 66% with osteoarthritis) demonstrated a 5.6% revision rate at a similar mean follow-up of 3.5 years. However, this study demonstrated that patients with a surface arthroplasty risk index (SARI) less than or equal to 3 had a 97% survivorship, and those with a SARI greater than 3 were 4.2 times more likely to require revision (see Table 2). In addition, 54% to 72% had high activity scores after hip resurfacing in 2 studies, 1 a randomized clinical trial.[62,63] An increase in participation in sports after hip resurfacing arthroplasty has also been seen in 2 questionnaire-based studies.[64,65] A randomized trail in the French literature comparing 71 THAs and 81 hip resurfacing arthroplasties demonstrated that the mean intensity of sport after surgery was higher in the resurfacing group, but the difference was smaller than previously demonstrated.[66]

Pathologic conditions increase the revision rate and are most likely more amenable to THA than hip resurfacing arthroplasty. Patients with osteonecrosis of the femoral head in retrospective analysis of 73 and 42 hip resurfacing arthroplasties at 5- and 4-years mean follow-up, respectively, show an increased revision rate of 7% when compared with hip resurfacing arthroplasty for osteoarthritis (see Table 2).[67,68] The Australian Orthopaedic Association National Joint Replacement Registry supports these findings and has increased revision rates for other pathologic conditions such as inflammatory arthritis and developmental dysplasia of the hip with hip resurfacing arthroplasty. Despite these results, there is a small series of 42 hip resurfacing arthroplasties with a survivorship of 97.6% at a mean of 3 years, which has demonstrated some success in this patient population.[69]

COMPLICATIONS AND CONCERNS

Femoral neck fracture is a complication that is not present in THA and that is unique to resurfacing arthroplasty (Table 3). The incidence of femoral neck fracture in metal-on-metal hip resurfacing

Table 3
Established risks of hip resurfacing arthroplasty and their corresponding highest level of evidence

Risk	Evidence	Citations
The incidence of femoral neck fracture in modern hip resurfacing arthroplasty is between 0% and 2%	Level IV, B	60,70
Women and patients who are obese have a higher risk of femoral neck fracture with hip resurfacing arthroplasty	Level II, B	33,71,72
Femoral neck notching and varus femoral component placement are associated with a femoral neck fracture	Level IV, B	33
Femoral neck fracture rate is subject to a surgical learning curve	Level II, B	71
Weight bearing restrictions postoperatively	Level V, B	74,75
Cobalt and chromium metal ion levels are elevated and proportional to bearing diameter in metal-on-metal hip resurfacing arthroplasty	Level IV, B	76
Metal ions cross the placenta	Level III, B	82
No increase in cancer risk with metal-on-metal articulation	Level III, B	83
Metal hypersensitivity may contribute to early osteolysis	Level IV, B	86
The formation of pseudotumors is suggestive of metal hypersensitivity	Level IV, B	90,91

Level of evidence Data from the Journal of Bone and Joint Surgery (I–IV) and the Orthopedic Clinics of North America (A or B); with permission.

arthroplasty ranges from 0% to 2.4% in various retrospective studies, which represents a marked improvement from the 7% to 12% fracture rate seen with metal-on-polyethylene implants.[16,34,60,70] A large retrospective review of 3429 metal-on-metal hip resurfacing arthroplasties found a femoral neck fracture rate of 1.46% at a mean of 15 weeks. In addition, women were more than twice as likely as men to have a femoral neck fracture, even though women fractured almost 5 weeks later (at 18.5 weeks) and had prodromal symptoms of pain and limping. Technical issues, including femoral neck notching and varus positioning of the femoral component, were present in 85% of the 50 hip fractures in this study (see **Table 3**).[33] Consequently, conversion to THA is recommended if these issues are noticed intraoperatively. A prospective cohort study of 550 hip resurfacing arthroplasties found that the femoral neck fracture rate was 8 times higher in the first 69 hip resurfacing arthroplasties but that the incidence was reduced to 0.4% after that time point, suggesting that this complication was linked to a surgical learning curve. In addition, women and patients who were obese (ie, body mass index >35) were over 3 times more likely to sustain a femoral neck fracture (see **Table 3**).[71] In fact, modification of the inclusion criteria in a prospective evaluation of hip resurfacing arthroplasty to exclude patients with osteopenia, obesity, or cysts greater that 1 cm in the femoral head reduced the overall complication rate from 13.4% to 2.1% and decreased the rate of femoral neck fracture from 7.2% to 0.8%.[72] Nondisplaced femoral neck fractures for as long as 4 months postoperatively have been successfully treated nonoperatively with restricted weight bearing, with 100% union in 7 patients.[73] Based on this observation and retrieval studies showing failure of bone healing at the neck-implant interface in failed hip resurfacing arthroplasty, an initial period of restricted weight bearing is recommended (see **Table 3**).[74,75]

One of the most debated and contentious concern, not specific to hip resurfacing arthroplasty, is that metal ion is released from metal-on-metal bearing surface wear. Mean serum chrome and cobalt levels are elevated in patients with metal-on-metal hip resurfacing arthroplasties (38 and 53 nmol/L, respectively) when compared with the upper limit of normal for each metal ion (5 nmol/L) in the population.[76] These changes in metal ion concentrations persist and have been documented for as long as 52 months postimplantation.[77,78] In addition, the diameter of a metal-on-metal bearing is proportional to level of metal ions released (see **Table 3**).[76] The exact level of metal ions required for a pathologic response is difficult to determine.[79] Patients with cobalt-chromium articulations have as high as a 2.5-fold increase in aneuploidy and 3.5-fold increase in chromosomal translocations in peripheral blood lymphocytes when compared with those with other articulations.[80,81] The unknown long-term ramifications of these elevated levels of ions and evidence that cobalt and chromium ions pass placental barrier prompt the recommendation that women of childbearing age should consider other bearing surfaces (see **Table 3**).[82] Although this metal-on-metal bearing surface change has helped reduce the occurrence of osteolysis, it has raised concern regarding circulating metal ion concentrations no matter how small and despite meta-analysis data demonstrating no increased risk of cancer after metal-on-metal THA (see **Table 3**).[83]

Metal hypersensitivity has been proposed as a mechanism for hip resurfacing arthroplasty loosening and osteolysis. Symptoms of metal hypersensitivity include unexplained groin pain, large joint effusion, and periprosthetic osteolysis approximately 2 years postimplantation.[84,85] Retrospective evaluation of resurfacing arthroplasties revealed a positive cobalt hypersensitivity test associated with early osteolysis, and periprosthetic tissue isolated at revision showed particle-laden macrophages and a lymphocytic infiltrate consistent with osteolysis (see **Table 3**).[86,87] Elevated peripheral blood lymphocyte activity to metal ion stimulation has been observed in patients undergoing revision of failed metal-on-metal implants. This reaction is consistent with type IV delayed hypersensitivity response.[88] Hypersensitivity may develop in previously unresponsive patients, making screening difficult.[89] The formation of pseudotumors in patients also supports the development of type IV delayed hypersensitivity response to metal debris (see **Table 3**).[90,91]

SUMMARY

The choice of arthroplasty technology should be individualized for each patient based on the relative risks and benefits of the device. However, decision making is often complicated by an increasing array of implant choices and a lack of long-term data on many implant systems. Until long-term clinical evidence for alternate bearing surfaces (eg, metal and ceramic) and hip resurfacing arthroplasty is available, there will be many questions and concerns regarding hip resurfacing arthroplasty. Hip resurfacing arthroplasty when performed with optimal technique in the properly selected patient should improve outcomes and minimize complications.

REFERENCES

1. Schmalzried TP. Why total hip resurfacing. J Arthroplasty 2007;22(7 Suppl 3):57–60.
2. Howie DW, Cornish BL, Vernon-Roberts B. Resurfacing hip arthroplasty. Classification of loosening and the role of prosthesis wear particles. Clin Orthop Relat Res 1990;255:144–59.
3. Amstutz HC, Campbell P, Kossovsky N, et al. Mechanism and clinical significance of wear debris-induced osteolysis. Clin Orthop Relat Res 1992; 276:7–18.
4. Grigoris P, Roberts P, Panousis K, et al. Hip resurfacing arthroplasty: the evolution of contemporary designs. Proc Inst Mech Eng H 2006;220(2): 95–105.
5. Kabo JM, Gebhard JS, Loren G, et al. In vivo wear of polyethylene acetabular components. J Bone Joint Surg Br 1993;75(2):254–8.
6. Chan FW, Bobyn JD, Medley JB, et al. Engineering issues and wear performance of metal on metal hip implants. Clin Orthop Relat Res 1996;333: 96–107.
7. Dowson D, Hardaker C, Flett M, et al. A hip joint simulator study of the performance of metal-on-metal joints: part II: design. J Arthroplasty 2004; 19(8 Suppl 3):124–30.
8. Rieker CB, Schon R, Konrad R, et al. Influence of the clearance on in-vitro tribology of large diameter metal-on-metal articulations pertaining to resurfacing hip implants. Orthop Clin North Am 2005;36(2): 135–42, vii.
9. Isaac GH, Siebel T, Schmalzried TP, et al. Development rationale for an articular surface replacement: a science-based evolution. Proc Inst Mech Eng H 2006;220(2):253–68.
10. Lin ZM, Meakins S, Morlock MM, et al. Deformation of press-fitted metallic resurfacing cups. Part 1: experimental simulation. Proc Inst Mech Eng H 2006;220(2):299–309.
11. Yew A, Jin ZM, Donn A, et al. Deformation of press-fitted metallic resurfacing cups. Part 2: finite element simulation. Proc Inst Mech Eng H 2006; 220(2):311–9.
12. Campbell P, Beaule PE, Ebramzadeh E, et al. The John Charnley Award: a study of implant failure in metal-on-metal surface arthroplasties. Clin Orthop Relat Res 2006;453:35–46.
13. Gill HS, Campbell PA, Murray DW, et al. Reduction of the potential for thermal damage during hip resurfacing. J Bone Joint Surg Br 2007;89(1):16–20.
14. Mjoberg B. Loosening of the cemented hip prosthesis. The importance of heat injury. Acta Orthop Scand Suppl 1986;221:1–40.
15. Morlock MM, Bishop N, Ruther W, et al. Biomechanical, morphological, and histological analysis of early failures in hip resurfacing arthroplasty. Proc Inst Mech Eng H 2006;220(2):333–44.
16. Capello WN, Ireland PH, Trammell TR, et al. Conservative total hip arthroplasty: a procedure to conserve bone stock. Part I: analysis of sixty-six patients. Part II: analysis of failures. Clin Orthop Relat Res 1978; 134:59–74.
17. Amstutz HC, Graff-Radford A, Mai LL, et al. Surface replacement of the hip with the Tharies system. Two to five-year results. J Bone Joint Surg Am 1981; 63(7):1069–77.
18. Freeman MA, Bradley GW. ICLH double cup arthroplasty. Orthop Clin North Am 1982;13(4): 799–811.
19. Head WC. The Wagner surface replacement arthroplasty. Orthop Clin North Am 1982;13(4):789–97.
20. McBryde CW, Revell MP, Thomas AM, et al. The influence of surgical approach on outcome in Birmingham hip resurfacing. Clin Orthop Relat Res 2008;466(4):920–6.
21. Myers GJ, Morgan D, McBryde CW, et al. Does surgical approach influence component positioning with Birmingham Hip Resurfacing? Int Orthop 2009;33(1):59–63.
22. Steffen R, O'Rourke K, Gill HS, et al. The anterolateral approach leads to less disruption of the femoral head-neck blood supply than the posterior approach during hip resurfacing. J Bone Joint Surg Br 2007;89(10):1293–8.
23. Steffen RT, Smith SR, Urban JP, et al. The effect of hip resurfacing on oxygen concentration in the femoral head. J Bone Joint Surg Br 2005;87(11):1468–74.
24. Ganz R, Gill TJ, Gautier E, et al. Surgical dislocation of the adult hip a technique with full access to the femoral head and acetabulum without the risk of avascular necrosis. J Bone Joint Surg Br 2001; 83(8):1119–24.
25. Nork SE, Schar M, Pfander G, et al. Anatomic considerations for the choice of surgical approach for hip resurfacing arthroplasty. Orthop Clin North Am 2005;36(2):163–70, viii.
26. Little CP, Ruiz AL, Harding IJ, et al. Osteonecrosis in retrieved femoral heads after failed resurfacing arthroplasty of the hip. J Bone Joint Surg Br 2005; 87(3):320–3.
27. Beaule PE, Campbell P, Shim P. Femoral head blood flow during hip resurfacing. Clin Orthop Relat Res 2007;456:148–52.
28. Lavigne M, Kalhor M, Beck M, et al. Distribution of vascular foramina around the femoral head and neck junction: relevance for conservative intracapsular procedures of the hip. Orthop Clin North Am 2005;36(2):171–6, viii.
29. Beaule PE, Campbell PA, Hoke R, et al. Notching of the femoral neck during resurfacing arthroplasty of

the hip: a vascular study. J Bone Joint Surg Br 2006;
88(1):35–9.

30. de Waal Malefijt MC, Huiskes R. A clinical, radiological and biomechanical study of the TARA hip prosthesis. Arch Orthop Trauma Surg 1993;112(5):220–5.

31. Mardones RM, Gonzalez C, Chen Q, et al. Surgical treatment of femoroacetabular impingement: evaluation of the effect of the size of the resection. Surgical technique. J Bone Joint Surg Am 2006;88(Suppl 1 Pt 1):84–91.

32. Markolf KL, Amstutz HC. Mechanical strength of the femur following resurfacing and conventional total hip replacement procedures. Clin Orthop Relat Res 1980;147:170–80.

33. Shimmin AJ, Back D. Femoral neck fractures following Birmingham hip resurfacing: a national review of 50 cases. J Bone Joint Surg Br 2005; 87(4):463–4.

34. Freeman MA. Some anatomical and mechanical considerations relevant to the surface replacement of the femoral head. Clin Orthop Relat Res 1978; 134:19–24.

35. Beaule PE, Lee JL, Le Duff MJ, et al. Orientation of the femoral component in surface arthroplasty of the hip. A biomechanical and clinical analysis. J Bone Joint Surg Am 2004;86(9):2015–21.

36. Long JP, Bartel DL. Surgical variables affect the mechanics of a hip resurfacing system. Clin Orthop Relat Res 2006;453:115–22.

37. Radcliffe IA, Taylor M. Investigation into the effect of varus-valgus orientation on load transfer in the resurfaced femoral head: a multi-femur finite element analysis. Clin Biomech (Bristol, Avon) 2007;22(7):780–6.

38. Anglin C, Masri BA, Tonetti J, et al. Hip resurfacing femoral neck fracture influenced by valgus placement. Clin Orthop Relat Res 2007;465:71–9.

39. Silva M, Lee KH, Heisel C, et al. The biomechanical results of total hip resurfacing arthroplasty. J Bone Joint Surg Am 2004;86(1):40–6.

40. Loughead JM, Chesney D, Holland JP, et al. Comparison of offset in Birmingham hip resurfacing and hybrid total hip arthroplasty. J Bone Joint Surg Br 2005;87(2):163–6.

41. Girard J, Lavigne M, Vendittoli PA, et al. Biomechanical reconstruction of the hip: a randomised study comparing total hip resurfacing and total hip arthroplasty. J Bone Joint Surg Br 2006;88(6):721–6.

42. Vendittoli PA, Lavigne M, Girard J, et al. A randomised study comparing resection of acetabular bone at resurfacing and total hip replacement. J Bone Joint Surg Br 2006;88(8):997–1002.

43. Liu F, Leslie I, Williams S, et al. Development of computational wear simulation of metal-on-metal hip resurfacing replacements. J Biomech 2008; 41(3):686–94.

44. Thomas BJ, Amstutz HC. Revision surgery for failed surface arthroplasty of the hip. Clin Orthop Relat Res 1982;170:42–9.

45. Beaule PE, Dorey FJ, LeDuff M, et al. Risk factors affecting outcome of metal-on-metal surface arthroplasty of the hip. Clin Orthop Relat Res 2004;418:87–93.

46. Ball ST, Le Duff MJ, Amstutz HC. Early results of conversion of a failed femoral component in hip resurfacing arthroplasty. J Bone Joint Surg Am 2007; 89(4):735–41.

47. McGrath MS, Desser DR, Ulrich SD, et al. Total hip resurfacing in patients who are sixty years of age or older. J Bone Joint Surg Am 2008;90(Suppl 3):27–31.

48. Martini F, Lebherz C, Mayer F, et al. Precision of the measurements of periprosthetic bone mineral density in hips with a custom-made femoral stem. J Bone Joint Surg Br 2000;82(7):1065–71.

49. Kishida Y, Sugano N, Nishii T, et al. Preservation of the bone mineral density of the femur after surface replacement of the hip. J Bone Joint Surg Br 2004; 86(2):185–9.

50. Hing CB, Young DA, Dalziel RE, et al. Narrowing of the neck in resurfacing arthroplasty of the hip: a radiological study. J Bone Joint Surg Br 2007; 89(8):1019–24.

51. Vail TP, Mina CA, Yergler JD, et al. Metal-on-metal hip resurfacing compares favorably with THA at 2 years followup. Clin Orthop Relat Res 2006;453:123–31.

52. Pollard TC, Baker RP, Eastaugh-Waring SJ, et al. Treatment of the young active patient with osteoarthritis of the hip. A five- to seven-year comparison of hybrid total hip arthroplasty and metal-on-metal resurfacing. J Bone Joint Surg Br 2006;88(5):592–600.

53. Buergi ML, Walter WL. Hip resurfacing arthroplasty: the Australian experience. J Arthroplasty 2007;22(7 Suppl 3):61–5.

54. Stulberg BN, Fitts SM, Bowen AR, et al. Early return to function after hip resurfacing is it better than contemporary total hip arthroplasty? J Arthroplasty Jul 28 2009. [Epub ahead of print].

55. Mont MA, Seyler TM, Ragland PS, et al. Gait analysis of patients with resurfacing hip arthroplasty compared with hip osteoarthritis and standard total hip arthroplasty. J Arthroplasty 2007;22(1):100–8.

56. Lavigne M, Therrien M, Nantel J, et al. The John Charnley Award: the functional outcome of hip resurfacing and large-head THA is the same: a randomized, Double-blind Study. Clin Orthop Relat Res 2010;468(2):326–36.

57. Back DL, Smith JD, Dalziel RE, et al. Incidence of heterotopic ossification after hip resurfacing. ANZ J Surg 2007;77(8):642–7.

58. Hing CB, Back DL, Bailey M, et al. The results of primary Birmingham hip resurfacings at a mean of

five years. An independent prospective review of the first 230 hips. J Bone Joint Surg Br 2007;89(11): 1431–8.

59. Schmalzried TP, Silva M, de la Rosa MA, et al. Optimizing patient selection and outcomes with total hip resurfacing. Clin Orthop Relat Res 2005;441:200–4.

60. Daniel J, Pynsent PB, McMinn DJ. Metal-on-metal resurfacing of the hip in patients under the age of 55 years with osteoarthritis. J Bone Joint Surg Br 2004;86(2):177–84.

61. Treacy RB, McBryde CW, Pynsent PB. Birmingham hip resurfacing arthroplasty. A minimum follow-up of five years. J Bone Joint Surg Br 2005;87(2):167–70.

62. Amstutz HC, Beaule PE, Dorey FJ, et al. Metal-on-metal hybrid surface arthroplasty: two to six-year follow-up study. J Bone Joint Surg Am 2004;86(1): 28–39.

63. Vendittoli PA, Lavigne M, Roy AG, et al. A prospective randomized clinical trial comparing metal-on-metal total hip arthroplasty and metal-on-metal total hip resurfacing in patients less than 65 years old. Hip Int 2006;16(Suppl 4):73–81.

64. Narvani AA, Tsiridis E, Nwaboku HC, et al. Sporting activity following Birmingham hip resurfacing. Int J Sports Med 2006;27(6):505–7.

65. Naal FD, Maffiuletti NA, Munzinger U, et al. Sports after hip resurfacing arthroplasty. Am J Sports Med 2007;35(5):705–11.

66. Lavigne M, Masse V, Girard J, et al. [Return to sport after hip resurfacing or total hip arthroplasty: a randomized study]. Rev Chir Orthop Reparatrice Appar Mot 2008;94(4):361–7 [in French].

67. Beaule PE, Amstutz HC, Le Duff M, et al. Surface arthroplasty for osteonecrosis of the hip: hemiresurfacing versus metal-on-metal hybrid resurfacing. J Arthroplasty 2004;19(8 Suppl 3):54–8.

68. Revell MP, McBryde CW, Bhatnagar S, et al. Metal-on-metal hip resurfacing in osteonecrosis of the femoral head. J Bone Joint Surg Am 2006;88(Suppl 3):98–103.

69. Mont MA, Seyler TM, Marker DR, et al. Use of metal-on-metal total hip resurfacing for the treatment of osteonecrosis of the femoral head. J Bone Joint Surg Am 2006;88(Suppl 3):90–7.

70. Beaule PE, Le Duff M, Campbell P, et al. Metal-on-metal surface arthroplasty with a cemented femoral component: a 7-10 year follow-up study. J Arthroplasty 2004;19(8 Suppl 3):17–22.

71. Marker DR, Seyler TM, Jinnah RH, et al. Femoral neck fractures after metal-on-metal total hip resurfacing: a prospective cohort study. J Arthroplasty 2007;22(7 Suppl 3):66–71.

72. Mont MA, Seyler TM, Ulrich SD, et al. Effect of changing indications and techniques on total hip resurfacing. Clin Orthop Relat Res 2007;465:63–70.

73. Cossey AJ, Back DL, Shimmin A, et al. The nonoperative management of periprosthetic fractures

associated with the Birmingham hip resurfacing procedure. J Arthroplasty 2005;20(3):358–61.

74. Shimmin AJ, Bare J, Back DL. Complications associated with hip resurfacing arthroplasty. Orthop Clin North Am 2005;36(2):187–93, ix.

75. Shimmin A, Beaule PE, Campbell P. Metal-on-metal hip resurfacing arthroplasty. J Bone Joint Surg Am 2008;90(3):637–54.

76. Clarke MT, Lee PT, Arora A, et al. Levels of metal ions after small- and large-diameter metal-on-metal hip arthroplasty. J Bone Joint Surg Br 2003;85(6):913–7.

77. Brodner W, Bitzan P, Meisinger V, et al. Serum cobalt levels after metal-on-metal total hip arthroplasty. J Bone Joint Surg Am 2003;85(11):2168–73.

78. Savarino L, Granchi D, Ciapetti G, et al. Ion release in stable hip arthroplasties using metal-on-metal articulating surfaces: a comparison between short- and medium-term results. J Biomed Mater Res A 2003;66(3):450–6.

79. MacDonald SJ. Can a safe level for metal ions in patients with metal-on-metal total hip arthroplasties be determined? J Arthroplasty 2004;19(8 Suppl 3): 71–7.

80. Doherty AT, Howell RT, Ellis LA, et al. Increased chromosome translocations and aneuploidy in peripheral blood lymphocytes of patients having revision arthroplasty of the hip. J Bone Joint Surg Br 2001;83(7):1075–81.

81. Ladon D, Doherty A, Newson R, et al. Changes in metal levels and chromosome aberrations in the peripheral blood of patients after metal-on-metal hip arthroplasty. J Arthroplasty 2004;19(8 Suppl 3): 78–83.

82. Ziaee H, Daniel J, Datta AK, et al. Transplacental transfer of cobalt and chromium in patients with metal-on-metal hip arthroplasty: a controlled study. J Bone Joint Surg Br 2007;89(3):301–5.

83. Tharani R, Dorey FJ, Schmalzried TP. The risk of cancer following total hip or knee arthroplasty. J Bone Joint Surg Am 2001;83(5):774–80.

84. Al-Saffar N. Early clinical failure of total joint replacement in association with follicular proliferation of B-lymphocytes: a report of two cases. J Bone Joint Surg Am 2002;84(12):2270–3.

85. Campbell P, Shimmin A, Walter L, et al. Metal sensitivity as a cause of groin pain in metal-on-metal hip resurfacing. J Arthroplasty 2008;23(7):1080–5.

86. Park YS, Moon YW, Lim SJ, et al. Early osteolysis following second-generation metal-on-metal hip replacement. J Bone Joint Surg Am 2005;87(7): 1515–21.

87. Witzleb WC, Hanisch U, Kolar N, et al. Neo-capsule tissue reactions in metal-on-metal hip arthroplasty. Acta Orthop 2007;78(2):211–20.

88. Christiansen K, Holmes K, Zilko PJ. Metal sensitivity causing loosened joint prostheses. Ann Rheum Dis 1980;39(5):476–80.

89. Merritt K, Rodrigo JJ. Immune response to synthetic materials. Sensitization of patients receiving orthopaedic implants. Clin Orthop Relat Res 1996;326: 71–9.

90. Pandit H, Glyn-Jones S, McLardy-Smith P, et al. Pseudotumours associated with metal-on-metal hip resurfacings. J Bone Joint Surg Br 2008;90(7): 847–51.

91. Pandit H, Vlychou M, Whitwell D, et al. Necrotic granulomatous pseudotumours in bilateral resurfacing hip arthroplasties: evidence for a type IV immune response. Virchows Arch 2008;453(5):529–34.

DVT Prophylaxis in Total Joint Reconstruction

Neil P. Sheth, MD[a], Jay R. Lieberman, MD[b],*,
Craig J. Della Valle, MD[c]

KEYWORDS
- Prophylaxis • Deep venous thrombosis
- Venous thromboembolism • Total joint arthroplasty

Deep venous thrombosis (DVT) is the end result of a complex interaction of events including the activation of the clotting cascade in conjunction with platelet aggregation. It has been clearly demonstrated that patients undergoing major lower extremity orthopedic surgery, especially total joint arthroplasty (TJA), are at high risk for developing a postoperative DVT or a subsequent pulmonary embolus (PE). In the arena of TJA, orthopedic surgeons are particularly concerned with proximal DVT and symptomatic or fatal PE.

Patients undergoing primary total hip arthroplasty (THA) or total knee arthroplasty (TKA) have exhibited rates of symptomatic PE as high as 20% and 8%, respectively when no prophylaxis has been administered.[1] As a result, the use of venous thromboembolic (DVT and PE) prophylaxis, most commonly pharmacologic prophylaxis, has become the standard of care for patients undergoing elective TJA. The risk of fatal PE following primary hip or knee replacement has been consistently reported to be between 0.1% and 0.2%, regardless of the chemoprophylactic agent employed for prophylaxis.[2–9]

Based on the necessity of postoperative venous thromboembolic (VTE) prophylaxis following TJA, the National Quality Forum endorsed a voluntary consensus standard for inpatient hospital care in the earlier part of this decade. The surgical care improvement project (SCIP) guidelines, a result of the consensus, require documentation of initiation of DVT prophylaxis in the time period extending from 24 hours before surgery to 24 hours following surgery.[10] The rationale for the SCIP guidelines stemmed from the government's emphasis on pay-for-performance (P4P) whereby physicians receive increased compensation as a function of meeting certain "standards of care."[11]

Despite several years of evaluating this question, the best prophylaxis for thromboembolic disease remains controversial.[12] The use of pharmacologic prophylaxis has been adopted as the standard of care for treatment of these patients by many orthopedic surgeons at most centers across North America.[13] However, the controversy between the efficacy of VTE prophylaxis and the increased risk for bleeding in the postoperative period continues to exist. In recent years, this debate has brought about the development of clinical guidelines to improve patient care, address key questions, define evidence-based recommendations, and promote future research. Clinical guidelines are not meant to represent a predefined protocol or absolute rules for treatment, and should never substitute for clinical judgment.

The authors have not received any financial support for the work and have no other financial or personal connections to the work presented in this article.

[a] Department of Orthopaedic Surgery, Rush University, Midwest Orthopaedics, 1725 West Harrison Street, Chicago, IL 60612, USA
[b] Department of Orthopaedic Surgery, New England Musculoskeletal Institute, Medical Arts and Research Building, University of Connecticut Health Center, 263 Farmington Avenue, Farmington, CT 06030-4038, USA
[c] Department of Orthopaedic Surgery, Rush University, 1725 West Harrison Street, Chicago, IL 60612, USA
* Corresponding author.
E-mail address: JLieberman@uchc.edu

Dependent on the clinical guideline followed, from the American College of Chest Physicians (ACCP) or the American Academy of Orthopaedic Surgeons (AAOS), there are several recommended regimens available for treatment. Included in the options are low molecular weight heparins (LMWHs), synthetic pentasaccharides, adjusted-dose warfarin, aspirin, and mechanical prophylaxis. Several studies have evaluated the various modalities for DVT prophylaxis, and comparison studies have stratified the risks and benefits for each option.

The following review addresses the controversy underlying VTE prophylaxis by outlining 2 guidelines and demonstrating the pros and cons of different DVT prophylaxis regimens based on the available evidence-based literature.

AMERICAN COLLEGE OF CHEST PHYSICIANS GUIDELINES

The ACCP was founded in 1935, and the first set of guidelines for venous thromboembolic prophylaxis (VTE) was published in 1986. The goal of these guidelines is to focus on the prevention of the overall rate of VTE. These guidelines are based on a review of prospective, randomized studies only. The guidelines have subsequently gone through several iterations with the most recent update in 2008.[13] Inherent to these guidelines is that all primary THA and TKA patients are considered "high risk" regardless of patient age, activity level, and comorbidities.

These guidelines have become commonplace in the evaluation of health care systems on behalf of hospitals, insurance companies, and attorneys. The recommendations were classified as Grade I (strong recommendation, with benefits outweighing risk, burden, and cost) or Grade II (recommendation with less certainty). Each class of recommendation was further substratified: (A) randomized controlled trials with consistent results and a low level of bias, (B) randomized controlled trials with inconsistent results or a major methodological design flaw, and (C) observational studies.[13] The use of LMWH, fondaparinux (pentasaccharide), and warfarin (with an adjusted international normalized ratio [INR] between 2.0 and 3.0) all received a Grade IA recommendation for preventative treatment of total hip and knee arthroplasty; aspirin or low-dose unfractionated heparin received a Grade IA rating against their use for prophylaxis in patients following TJA. The use of intermittent pneumatic compression devices received a Grade IB rating for prevention in patients undergoing TKA.

These guidelines also address the duration of prophylaxis. During the first iteration, the ACCP guidelines from 1998 and 2001 recommended 7 to 10 days of prophylaxis that coincided with the length of hospital stay (Grade IA recommendation).[14] In 2004, the guidelines were revised to recommend out of hospital prophylaxis for 28 to 35 days (Grade IA) but excluded patients undergoing TKA.[15] With additional revisions, the 2008 guidelines currently recommend duration of prophylaxis with LMWH, fondaparinux, and warfarin for up to 10 days following THA and TKA (Grade IA), and up to 35 days following THA (Grade IA) or TKA (Grade IIB).[13]

As with any guidelines being used to guide physicians in medical decision making, the risk versus benefit must be assessed. Implementation of the current ACCP guidelines has been associated with certain disadvantages, as reported in the orthopedic literature. Burnett and colleagues[16] reported a 4.7% readmission rate, 3.4% irrigation and debridement rate, and 5.1% rate of prolonged hospitalization following 10 days of LMWH after TJA. Parvizi and colleagues[17] have shown that patients with a wound hematoma or persistent wound drainage are at higher risk for a postoperative deep joint infection. As a direct consequence of the concerns for postoperative bleeding risk and potential for infection, orthopedic surgeons may prefer a more risk-averse method by which to prevent thromboembolic phenomena following TJA, especially because the rate of PE is similar regardless of the chemoprophylaxis agent used.

AMERICAN ACADEMY OF ORTHOPEDIC SURGEONS GUIDELINES

A work group from the AAOS in conjunction with the Center for Clinical Evidence Synthesis (Tufts New England Medical Center) proposed a new set of guidelines for the prevention of symptomatic and fatal PE in patients undergoing elective TJA. The AAOS guidelines are a synthesis of an expert consensus as well as an analysis of 42 articles published since 1996, and focus on the prevention of symptomatic PE. The clinical outcomes of choice for evaluation included symptomatic and fatal PE, death, and major bleeding episodes following TJA.[18] Consensus recommendations included the use of regional anesthesia, mechanical prophylaxis for all patients, rapid postoperative mobilization, and adequate patient education. Each patient required a preoperative evaluation for a determination of "standard" and "high" risk potential. The choice of a specific chemoprophylaxis agent was based on the individual risk-benefit profile for PE and bleeding complication.

Each recommendation was graded using the following system: (A) good evidence (level I studies with consistent findings) for recommending intervention, (B) fair evidence (level II or III studies with consistent findings) for recommending intervention, and (C) poor-quality evidence (level IV or V) for recommending intervention[18] (**Table 1**). Of the total number of recommendations from this set of guidelines, only 4 of them were derived from a systematic review of the literature. Additional general consensus recommendations are listed in **Table 2**.[18]

For patients at standard risk for both PE and major bleeding complications, the recommendation is as follows: aspirin, LMWH, pentasaccharide, or warfarin (INR goal of ≤2.0). This recommendation is based on level III evidence and was given a grade of B or C.

For patients at elevated risk for PE and standard risk for major bleeding complications, the recommendation is as follows: LMWH, pentasaccharide, or warfarin (INR goal of ≤2.0). This recommendation is based on level III evidence and was given a grade of B or C.

For patients with standard risk of PE and elevated risk of major bleeding complications, the recommendation is as follows: aspirin, warfarin (INR goal of ≤2.0), or none. This recommendation is based on level III evidence and was given a grade of C.

For patients with elevated risk of both PE and major bleeding complications, the recommendation is as follows: aspirin, warfarin (INR goal of ≤2.0), or none. This recommendation is based on level III evidence and was given a grade of C.

The most important concept that is fundamental to the AAOS guidelines for thromboembolic prophylaxis is that the risk versus benefit for each individual patient must be assessed in the preoperative period. The general recommendations presented in **Table 2** are a result of the work group's consensus, and address a majority of the perioperative issues with prophylaxis. For patients with elevated risks for PE, major bleeding complication, or both, these guidelines provide an effective manner by which to treat these patients in the postoperative period following TJA. However,

a weakness inherent to the AAOS guidelines is the inability to accurately assess the preoperative risk for DVT/PE. In reality, based on the nature of TJA, arthroplasty patients may not truly be considered low risk. In addition, there are studies to demonstrate rates of VTE as high as 72% following the administration of aspirin,[19] thus raising the question of whether the use of aspirin is adequate as a thromboprophylaxis agent.

LOW MOLECULAR WEIGHT HEPARINS

The use of LMWH has gained enthusiasm within the orthopedic community due to its well-documented bioavailability and the absence of monitoring for clotting indices (ie, INR). The efficacy of LMWH is well documented. In multiple randomized trials, including THA and TKA patients, LMWH has been more effective than warfarin in limiting overall DVT rates. However, LMWH is associated with higher bleeding rates. Because the selection of a prophylaxis agent is a balance between efficacy and safety, some surgeons choose other modes of prophylaxis due to concerns related to bleeding and its impact on overall outcomes. An additional consideration with any medication choice is the cost; the cost of LMWH remains relatively high as compared with aspirin and warfarin.

As with any postoperative chemoprophylaxis regimen, duration of treatment is always of concern. The ACCP guidelines have changed their recommendations since the initial guidelines introduced in 1998. The most recent recommendation from the ACCP in 2008 states that patients undergoing THA or TKA should receive chemoprophylaxis with LMWH for 7 to 10 days (Grade IA recommendation), and this may be extended to up to 35 days following THA. Administration of LMWH for 35 days following TKA received a Grade 2B recommendation.[13] As stated previously, the choice of agent as well as the duration of prophylaxis is based on a risk versus benefit analysis which should be individualized for each arthroplasty patient.

FONDAPARINUX

Fondaparinux is a newer synthetic pentasaccharide that is a potent inhibitor of Factor Xa in the clotting cascade. The typical dosing is 2.5 mg/d administered subcutaneously with the first dose being given at 6 to 12 hours postoperatively. This drug is not recommended for patients that weigh less than 50 kg or those with renal insufficiency. As with LMWH, the concern associated with the use of fondaparinux is for bleeding complications in the postoperative period.[20]

Table 1 Levels of evidence	
Level I	High-quality randomized trial
Level II	Cohort study (good control)
Level III	Case-control study
Level IV	Uncontrolled case series
Level V	Expert opinion

Table 2
Consensus recommendations from the AAOS work group

General Recommendation	Level of Evidence	Grade
Assess all patients preoperatively with regard to their risk (standard vs high) of pulmonary embolism	Level III	Grade C
Assess all patients preoperatively with regard to their risk (standard vs high) of bleeding complications	Level III	Grade C
Consider vena cava filter placement for patients who have a known contraindication to anticoagulation therapy	Level V	Grade C
Consider intraoperative or immediate postoperative mechanical compression	Level III	Grade B
Consider regional anesthesia for the procedure (in consultation with anesthesia team)	Level IV	Grade C
Consider use of mechanical prophylaxis postoperatively	Level IV	Grade C
Rapid patient mobilization	Level V	Grade C
Routine screening for thromboembolism is not recommended	Level III	Grade B
Educate the patient about symptoms of thromboembolism	Level V	Grade B

Data from Johanson NA, Lachiewicz PF, Lieberman JR, et al. Prevention of symptomatic pulmonary embolism in patients undergoing total hip or knee arthroplasty. J Am Acad Orthop Surg 2009;17(3):183–96.

The use of fondaparinux received a Grade 1A recommendation from the ACCP for use in patients undergoing primary elective TJA. Regarding duration of treatment, the most recent changes to the ACCP guidelines in 2008 support the use of the agent for 35 days after THA (Grade 1A) and after TKA (Grade 1B).[13,21] There are concerns about using this drug in patients at an increased rate of bleeding as seen in the AAOS guidelines, but this is not an evidence-based recommendation.

WARFARIN

Warfarin is the oldest vitamin K antagonist used for chemoprophylaxis, with the longest track record of use in the postoperative period following primary hip or knee arthroplasty. The traditional nature of medicine has helped maintain warfarin as a popular agent, because it was the treatment of choice when most orthopedic surgeons trained during residency. Warfarin has demonstrated efficacy as an effective chemoprophylaxis agent against thromboembolic disease; however, it is not without its disadvantages. Immediately post administration, the patient is in a relatively hyper-coagulable state due to diminished levels of protein C and protein S via actions of the drug. Each patient requires daily dosing and the blood is monitored daily for an INR level to determine the appropriate dose to administer. Warfarin is very sensitive to dietary changes and has interactions with several medications that may be concomitantly taken by a patient for other comorbid conditions (**Table 3**). As a result, the goal INR is difficult to achieve and maintain.

A meta-analysis of all randomized controlled clinical trials reported on the overall efficacy of warfarin as a prophylactic agent following THA. Patients treated with warfarin had the lowest rate of proximal DVT as well as symptomatic PE, with a rate of 6.3% and 0.16%, respectively. The risk of major postoperative bleeding in these patients was no higher than that in patients treated with a placebo.[4]

The use of warfarin as an effective prophylactic agent following TKA has been thoroughly demonstrated over several decades.[22–26] Additional

Table 3
Common drug interactions with warfarin

Trimethoprim-sulfamethoxazole (Bactrim)
Rifampin
Macrolide antibiotics (ie, erythromycin)
Quinolone antibiotics (ie, ciprofloxacin)
Metronidazole (Flagyl)
Certain cephalosporins (cefamandole)
Thyroid hormones (ie, levothyroxine)
Phenytoin (Dilantin)
Cimetidine (Tagamet)
Anitarrhythmics (ie, amiodarone)
Herbal medications (ie, garlic)

randomized clinical trials have compared the efficacy of warfarin with that of LMWH.[24,26–29] In every study, LMWH was more effective than warfarin as a prophylactic agent, but there was no significant difference in the rates of symptomatic proximal DVT or PE. The postoperative bleeding rates were typically higher in the LMWH group.[24,26,29]

With regard to the goal INR, different clinical guidelines present differing recommendations. According to the ACCP clinical guideline, a goal INR of 2.0 to 3.0 received a Grade 1A recommendation. This recommendation was made based on randomized trials that used an INR range of 2.0 to 3.0 as the target for prophylaxis.[13] For each scenario depicted by the AAOS where the use of warfarin is warranted, the goal INR is 2.0 or less. The difference in the goal INR is based on risk versus benefit between prophylaxis against thromboembolic disease and bleeding risk. The AAOS guidelines consistently make recommendations that are more conservative and attempt to minimize the postoperative bleeding risk and hematoma formation.

As with the use of LMWH, the ACCP guidelines have changed their recommendations regarding the duration of warfarin use following primary hip or knee replacement. The 2008 ACCP guidelines recommend up to 35 days of warfarin use (goal INR 2.0–3.0) with a Grade 1B recommendation for THA and a Grade 1C recommendation for TKA patients. The AAOS recommendation, for patients of standard risk for PE and bleeding, is 2 to 6 weeks of treatment with low-dose warfarin (goal INR ≤2.0). Even in patients with an elevated PE and bleeding risk, low-dose warfarin is recommended for 2 to 6 weeks.

ASPIRIN

Acetylsalicylic acid (aspirin) has gained in popularity as an agent for DVT prophylaxis following total joint replacement because it is safe, inexpensive, does not require monitoring, is easy to administer, and lends itself to high patient compliance. The recommended dosing in the postoperative period is 325 mg twice daily for the duration of treatment.[18] The use of aspirin is based on the premise that chemoprophylaxis should be administered to reduce the risk of PE and subsequent death, not DVT; inherent to this argument is that DVT should not be used as a surrogate for PE because all patients with a DVT do not inevitably get a PE.

Aspirin does not interfere with anesthetic administration because it does not increase the risk of neuraxial bleeding. The use of an epidural catheter for pain control requires that postoperative chemoprophylaxis be timed appropriately to minimize the risk of epidural hematoma formation.[30] Aspirin functions by way of inhibiting platelet aggregation, and if given immediately preoperatively, can function in this manner intraoperatively and in the immediate postoperative period; other chemoprophylaxis agents exhibit a postoperative delay before the onset of the desired prophylaxis effect. The major benefit associated with aspirin use is its low prevalence of wound-healing problems, hematoma formation, and other serious bleeding complications that are readily associated with more potent anticoagulant agents.[31]

In the arena of TKA, aspirin has been equally as effective as other anticoagulant agents when fatal PE is used as an end point.[32] Lotke and colleagues[33] reported on 2800 consecutive primary TKAs in patients treated with aspirin and mechanical prophylaxis, demonstrating a low rate of bleeding complication and a fatal PE risk of 0.1%. However, aspirin is not as effective in decreasing the risk of symptomatic DVT in the setting of THA. The Pulmonary Embolism Prevention trial was a randomized clinical trial designed to evaluate the efficacy of aspirin in preventing symptomatic VTE disease following THA. More than 4000 patients were randomized to receive aspirin (n = 2047) or a placebo (n = 2041) for 35 days following surgery. There was no statistical difference in the rate of symptomatic DVT between the 2 groups ($P>.5$).

In general, venous thromboembolic events following primary hip and knee arthroplasty has decreased significantly over the past decade, mainly due to a multidisciplinary approach. Rapid postoperative mobilization, optimization of surgical technique, and improved perioperative pain management, including the use of regional anesthesia, have all contributed to decreasing the DVT risk. The ACCP guidelines do not support the use of aspirin for prophylaxis following TJA, because this drug has not been extensively evaluated in multicenter randomized trials. The AAOS guidelines support the use of aspirin for 6 weeks except in patients that are at high risk for PE and have standard bleeding complication risk; these patients are not candidates for aspirin use because of the identified preoperative elevated risk for PE.

Because the selection of a prophylaxis agent is a balance between safety and efficacy, aspirin combined with mechanical devices is an attractive regimen for some orthopedic surgeons for their routine TJA patients. Although aspirin is less potent than other chemoprophylactic agents, it is also associated with less bleeding. Aspirin needs to be evaluated in large randomized trials that assess symptomatic events to determine its true efficacy.

MECHANICAL PROPHYLAXIS (PNEUMATIC COMPRESSION BOOTS AND INTERMITTENT PLANTAR COMPRESSION DEVICES)

The use of mechanical prophylaxis is predicated on the premise that decreasing lower extremity venous stasis in conjunction with increasing venous blood flow will decrease the likelihood of clot formation.[34,35] Pneumatic compression boots affect local fibrinolysis, but do not affect systemic fibrinolytic activity.[36] Intermittent plantar compression devices were designed to replicate the hemodynamic effects of normal walking by rapid emptying of the plantar arch during the compression phase of the device.[12] The advantages of mechanical prophylaxis are evident and include an absence of monitoring and no risk of bleeding. In addition, intermittent plantar compression devices are thought to be less cumbersome than pneumatic boots, which extend the length of the entire lower leg. However, the major disadvantages are that prophylaxis ceases on patient discharge from the hospital, and patient compliance is critical to either device being effective.

Several randomized clinical trials have demonstrated that pneumatic compression boots can limit distal thrombus formation.[23,37–41] As a result, there has been concern regarding the efficacy of mechanical compression in reducing the rates of proximal clot formation in the setting of THA. Small randomized trials have compared pneumatic compression boots and warfarin in patients undergoing THA and have demonstrated that mechanical prophylaxis is less effective than chemoprophylaxis in the prevention of proximal clot formation.[39–41] Regarding intermittent plantar compression devices, low-powered studies have shown a decrease in overall thrombosis rates following THA.[42–44] However, given the risk of PE from a proximal clot source, further investigation is required before mechanical prophylaxis can be recommended as a sole means of prophylaxis in patients undergoing THA.

The use of mechanical prophylaxis in the setting of TKA, both pneumatic compression and intermittent plantar compression, has been studied in several small studies.[19,23,44–49] Although these studies were low powered, a significant reduction in thrombus formation following TKA was demonstrated. On basis of these reports, both pneumatic compression and intermittent plantar compression devices are effective in reducing clot formation following primary TKA. However, larger, multicenter randomized trials comparing mechanical and chemoprophylaxis regimens are necessary to determine the true efficacy of these devices.

AUTHORS' COMMENTARY ON CURRENT GUIDELINES

The basic difference between the ACCP and the AAOS guidelines is that the chest physicians believe that asymptomatic clots are clinically relevant. Therefore, the ACCP guidelines were developed from the data obtained from randomized trials, which used venogram data as a surrogate outcome measure. In contrast, the AAOS guidelines reflect the concerns of orthopedic surgeons with a focus on symptomatic clots, PE, and bleeding risk. Furthermore, the AAOS guidelines highlight the importance of developing prophylaxis regimens for each individual patient based on PE and bleeding risk. This is an important concept, which moves us toward risk stratification. Unfortunately, it is difficult to risk stratify most patients based on available data but it is a goal to strive for in the future.

Surgeons need to be aware that the SCIP guidelines recommend LMWH, fondaparinux, and/or warfarin for THA and TKA patients. Pneumatic compression devices are also acceptable for patients undergoing TKA procedures. Therefore, aspirin and pneumatic compression devices are acceptable for TKA patients. A surgeon may choose to use another regimen because of concerns about bleeding, but this must be documented in the medical record.

REFERENCES

1. Comp PC, Spiro TE, Friedman RJ, et al. Prolonged enoxaparin therapy to prevent venous thromboembolism after primary hip or knee replacement. Enoxaparin Clinical Trial Group. J Bone Joint Surg Am 2001;83(3):336–45.
2. Douketis JD, Eikelboom JW, Quinlan DJ, et al. Short-duration prophylaxis against venous thromboembolism after total hip or knee replacement: a meta-analysis of prospective studies investigating symptomatic outcomes. Arch Intern Med 2002; 162(13):1465–71.
3. Brookenthal KR, Freedman KB, Lotke PA, et al. A meta-analysis of thromboembolic prophylaxis in total knee arthroplasty. J Arthroplasty 2001;13(3): 293–300.
4. Freedman KB, Brookenthal KR, Fitzgerald RH Jr, et al. A meta-analysis of thromboembolic prophylaxis following elective total hip arthroplasty. J Bone Joint Surg Am 2000;82(7):929–38.
5. Larson CM, MacMillan DP, Lachiewicz PF. Thromboembolism after total knee arthroplasty: intermittent pneumatic compression and aspirin prophylaxis. J South Orthop Assoc 2001;10(3): 155–63 [discussion: 163].

6. Lieberman JR, Wollaeger J, Dorey F, et al. The efficacy of prophylaxis with low-dose warfarin for prevention of pulmonary embolism following total hip arthroplasty. J Bone Joint Surg Am 1997;79(3):319–25.

7. Nassif JM, Ritter MA, Meding JB, et al. The effect of intraoperative intravenous fixed-dose heparin during total joint arthroplasty on the incidence of fatal pulmonary emboli. J Arthroplasty 2000;15(1):16–21.

8. Sarmiento A, Goswami AD. Thromboembolic prophylaxis with use of aspirin, exercise, and graded elastic stockings or intermittent compression devices in patients managed with total hip arthroplasty. J Bone Joint Surg Am 1999;81(3):339–46.

9. Westrich GH, Haas SB, Mosca P, et al. Meta-analysis of thromboembolic prophylaxis after total knee arthroplasty. J Bone Joint Surg Br 2000;82(6):795–800.

10. SCIP guidelines. Available at: www.ashp.org. Accessed January 31, 2010.

11. Deitelzweig DW, Lin J, Hussein M, et al. Are surgical patients at risk of venous thromboembolism currently meeting the Surgical Care Improvement Project performance measure for appropriate and timely prophylaxis? J Thromb Thrombolysis 2009. [Epub ahead of print].

12. Lieberman JR, Hsu WK. Prevention of venous thromboembolic disease after total hip and knee arthroplasty. J Bone Joint Surg Am 2005;87(9):2097–112.

13. Geerts WH, Bergqvist D, Pineo GF, et al. Prevention of venous thromboembolism: American College of Chest Physicians Evidence-Based Clinical Practice Guidelines (8th Edition). Chest 2008;133(Suppl 6):381S–453S.

14. Geerts WH, Heit JA, Clagett GP, et al. Prevention of venous thromboembolism. Chest 2001;119(Suppl 1):132S–75S.

15. Geerts WH, Pineo GF, Heit JA, et al. Prevention of venous thromboembolism: the Seventh ACCP Conference on Antithrombotic and Thrombolytic Therapy. Chest 2004;126(Suppl 3):338S–400S.

16. Burnett RS, Clohisy JC, Wright RW, et al. Failure of the American College of Chest Physicians-1A protocol for lovenox in clinical outcomes for thromboembolic prophylaxis. J Arthroplasty 2007;22(3):317–24.

17. Parvizi J, Ghanem E, Joshi A, et al. Does "excessive" anticoagulation predispose to periprosthetic infection? J Arthroplasty 2007;22(6 Suppl 2):24–8.

18. Johanson NA, Lachiewicz PF, Lieberman JR, et al. Prevention of symptomatic pulmonary embolism in patients undergoing total hip or knee arthroplasty. J Am Acad Orthop Surg 2009;17(3):183–96.

19. Westrich GH, Sculco TP. Prophylaxis against deep venous thrombosis after total knee arthroplasty. Pneumatic plantar compression and aspirin compared with aspirin alone. J Bone Joint Surg Am 1996;78(6):826–34.

20. Turpie AG, Eriksson BI, Bauer KA, et al. Fondaparinux. J Am Acad Orthop Surg 2004;12(6):371–5.

21. Muntz J. Thromboprophylaxis in orthopedic surgery: how long is long enough? Am J Orthop 2009;38(8):394–401.

22. Robinson KS, Anderson DR, Gross M, et al. Ultrasonographic screening before hospital discharge for deep venous thrombosis after arthroplasty: the post-arthroplasty screening study. A randomized, controlled trial. Ann Intern Med 1997;127(6):439–45.

23. Kaempffe FA, Lifeso RM, Meinking C. Intermittent pneumatic compression versus coumadin. Prevention of deep vein thrombosis in lower-extremity total joint arthroplasty. Clin Orthop Relat Res 1991;269:89–97.

24. Fitzgerald RH Jr, Spiro TE, Trowbridge AA, et al. Prevention of venous thromboembolic disease following primary total knee arthroplasty. A randomized, multicenter, open-label, parallel-group comparison of enoxaparin and warfarin. J Bone Joint Surg Am 2001;83(6):900–6.

25. Heit JA, Elliott CG, Trowbridge AA, et al. Ardeparin sodium for extended out-of-hospital prophylaxis against venous thromboembolism after total hip or knee replacement. A randomized, double-blind, placebo-controlled trial. Ann Intern Med 2000;132(11):853–61.

26. Leclerc JR, Geerts WH, Desjardins L, et al. Prevention of venous thromboembolism after knee arthroplasty. A randomized, double-blind trial comparing enoxaparin with warfarin. Ann Intern Med 1996;124(7):619–26.

27. Hull R, Raskob G, Pineo G, et al. A comparison of subcutaneous low-molecular-weight heparin with warfarin sodium for prophylaxis against deep-vein thrombosis after hip or knee implantation. N Engl J Med 1993;329(19):1370–6.

28. RD Heparin Arthroplasty Group. RD heparin compared with warfarin for prevention of venous thromboembolic disease following total hip or knee arthroplasty. J Bone Joint Surg Am 1994;76(8):1174–85.

29. Heit JA, Berkowitz SD, Bona R, et al. Efficacy and safety of low molecular weight heparin (ardeparin sodium) compared to warfarin for the prevention of venous thromboembolism after total knee replacement surgery: a double-blind, dose-ranging study. Ardeparin Arthroplasty Study Group. Thromb Haemost 1997;77(1):32–8.

30. Mantilla CB, Horlocker TT, Schroeder DR, et al. Risk factors for clinically relevant pulmonary embolism and deep venous thrombosis in patients undergoing primary hip or knee arthroplasty. Anesthesiology 2003;9(3):552–60 [discussion: 5A].

31. Sharrock NE, Gonzalez Della Valle A, Go G, et al. Potent anticoagulants are associated with a higher all-cause mortality rate after hip and knee arthroplasty. Clin Orthop Relat Res 2008;466:714–21.

32. Lotke PA, Lonner JH. Deep venous thrombosis prophylaxis: better living through chemistry—in opposition. J Arthroplasty 2005;20(4 Suppl 2):15–7.

33. Lotke PA, Palevsky H, Keenan AM, et al. Aspirin and warfarin for thromboembolic disease after total joint arthroplasty. Clin Orthop Relat Res 1996;324:251–8.

34. Weitz J, Michelsen J, Gold K, et al. Effects of intermittent pneumatic calf compression on postoperative thrombin and plasmin activity. Thromb Haemost 1986;56(2):198–201.

35. Allenby F, Boardman L, Pflug JJ, et al. Effects of external pneumatic intermittent compression on fibrinolysis in man. Lancet 1973;2(7843):1412–4.

36. Sharrock NE, Go G, Mineo R, et al. The hemodynamic and fibrinolytic response to low dose epinephrine and phenylephrine infusions during total hip replacement under epidural anesthesia. Thromb Haemost 1992;68(4):436–41.

37. Hull RD, Raskob GE, Gent M, et al. Effectiveness of intermittent pneumatic leg compression for preventing deep vein thrombosis after total hip replacement. JAMA 1990;263(17):2313–7.

38. Gallus A, Raman K, Darby T. Venous thrombosis after elective hip replacement—the influence of preventive intermittent calf compression and of surgical technique. Br J Surg 1983;7(1):17–9.

39. Francis CW, Pellegrini VD Jr, Marder VJ, et al. Comparison of warfarin and external pneumatic compression in prevention of venous thrombosis after total hip replacement. JAMA 1992;267(21):2911–5.

40. Bailey JP, Kruger MP, Solano FX, et al. Prospective randomized trial of sequential compression devices vs low-dose warfarin for deep venous thrombosis prophylaxis in total hip arthroplasty. J Arthroplasty 1991;6(Suppl):S29–35.

41. Paiement G, Wessinger SJ, Waltman AC, et al. Low-dose warfarin versus external pneumatic compression for prophylaxis against venous thromboembolism following total hip replacement. J Arthroplasty 1987;2(1):23–6.

42. Fordyce MJ, Ling RS. A venous foot pump reduces thrombosis after total hip replacement. J Bone Joint Surg Br 1992;74(1):45–9.

43. Santori FS, Vitullo A, Stopponi M, et al. Prophylaxis against deep-vein thrombosis in total hip replacement. Comparison of heparin and foot impulse pump. J Bone Joint Surg Br 1994;76(4):579–83.

44. Warwick D, Harrison J, Glew D, et al. Comparison of the use of a foot pump with the use of low-molecular-weight heparin for the prevention of deep-vein thrombosis after total hip replacement. A prospective, randomized trial. J Bone Joint Surg Am 1998;80(8):1158–66.

45. Haas SB, Insall JN, Scuderi GR, et al. Pneumatic sequential-compression boots compared with aspirin prophylaxis of deep-vein thrombosis after total knee arthroplasty. J Bone Joint Surg Am 1990;72(1):27–31.

46. McKenna R, Galante J, Bachmann F, et al. Prevention of venous thromboembolism after total knee replacement by high-dose aspirin or intermittent calf and thigh compression. Br J Surg 1980;280(6213):514–7.

47. Hull R, Delmore TJ, Hirsh J, et al. Effectiveness of intermittent pulsatile elastic stockings for the prevention of calf and thigh vein thrombosis in patients undergoing elective knee surgery. Thromb Res 1979;16(1–2):37–45.

48. Blanchard J, Meuwly JY, Leyvraz PF, et al. Prevention of deep-vein thrombosis after total knee replacement. Randomised comparison between a low-molecular-weight heparin (nadroparin) and mechanical prophylaxis with a foot-pump system. J Bone Joint Surg Br 1999;81(4):654–9.

49. Tamir L, Hendel D, Neyman C, et al. Sequential foot compression reduces lower limb swelling and pain after total knee arthroplasty. J Arthroplasty 1999; 14(3):333–8.

Index

Note: Page numbers of article titles are in **boldface** type.

orthopedic.theclinics.com

Orthop Clin N Am 41 (2010) 281–285
doi:10.1016/S0030-5898(10)00024-6

Moving?

Make sure your subscription moves with you!

To notify us of your new address, find your **Clinics Account Number** (located on your mailing label above your name), and contact customer service at:

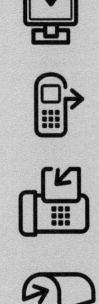

Email: journalscustomerservice-usa@elsevier.com

800-654-2452 (subscribers in the U.S. & Canada)
314-447-8871 (subscribers outside of the U.S. & Canada)

Fax number: 314-447-8029

Elsevier Health Sciences Division
Subscription Customer Service
3251 Riverport Lane
Maryland Heights, MO 63043

ELSEVIER

Printed and bound by CPI Group (UK) Ltd, Croydon, CR0 4YY

03/10/2024

01040360-0014